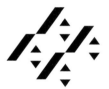

ATLAS

4

Learning-Centered
Communication

David Nunan

*with teacher's notes
by Fran Byrnes*

Heinle & Heinle Publishers
An International Thomson Publishing Company
Boston, MA 02116, U.S.A.

I(T)P   The ITP logo is a trademark under license.

The publication of ATLAS was directed by the
members of the Heinle & Heinle Global Innovations
Publishing Team:

Elizabeth Holthaus, ESL Team Leader
David C. Lee, Editorial Director
John F. McHugh, Market Development Director
Lisa McLaughlin, Production Editor
Nancy Mann, Developmental Editor

Also participating in the publication of the
program were:
Publisher: Stanley J. Galek
Assistant Editor: Kenneth Mattsson
Manufacturing Coordinator: Mary Beth Hennebury
Design and Production: Rollins Graphic Design and
Production
Composition: Pre-Press Company

Manufactured in the United States of America.

ISBN 0-8384-4096-7

Heinle & Heinle Publishers is an International
Thomson Publishing Company

10 9   8   7   6   5   4   3   2   1

Preface

Atlas is a four-level ESL/EFL course for young adults and adults. Its learner-centered, task-based approach motivates learners and helps to create an active, communicative classroom.

Atlas develops the four language skills of listening, speaking, reading, and writing in a systematic and integrated fashion. Each level is designed to cover from 60 to 90 hours of classroom instruction. It can also be adapted for shorter or longer courses; suggestions for doing so are provided in the teacher's extended edition.

Each level of Atlas consists of the following components:

Student's Book The student's book contains 12 "core" units and 3 review units. Following the 15 units are "Communication Challenges," which provide extra communicative practice to conclude each unit. Grammar summaries for each unit appear at the end of the book, along with an irregular verb chart.

Teacher's Extended Edition The teacher's extended edition contains an introduction to the philosophy of the course, general guidelines for teaching with Atlas, detailed teaching suggestions for each unit, and extension activities. It also includes the tapescript and answer keys for the textbook and the workbook.

Teacher Tape The tapes contain spoken material for all of the listening activities in the student text.

Workbook The workbook provides practice and expansion of the vocabulary, structures, functions, and learning strategies in the student text.

Workbook Tape The workbook tape contains spoken material for all of the listening activities in the workbook.

Video The video, which contains lively, real-life material, provides reinforcement and expansion of the topics and functions found in the student text.

Assessment Package The assessment package will be available in 1995.

FEATURES	BENEFITS
Unit goals are explicitly stated at the beginning of each unit.	Awareness of goals helps students to focus their learning.
Listening and reading texts are derived from high-interest, authentic source material.	Naturalistic/realistic language prepares students for the language they will encounter outside the classroom.
Each unit is built around two task chains, sequences of tasks that are linked together in principled ways and in which succeeding tasks are built on those that come before.	Task chains enhance student interest and motivation by providing students with integrated learning experiences.
Units feature explicit focus on learning strategies.	Conscious development of a range of learning strategies helps students become more effective learners both in and out of class.
End-of-unit Self-Check section encourages students to record and reflect on what they have learned.	Developing personal records of achievement increases student confidence and motivation.

Table of Contents

Language Focus Structures	Learning Strategies	Communication Challenges
• prepositional phrases • modals: *can/could/would/would mind*	• scanning* • selective listening • brainstorming • practicing • cooperating • personalizing	• Simulation: Planning a festival
• short responses • relative adverbials: *where/when/why/how*	• predicting* • making inferences • selective listening • evaluating • scanning • personalizing	• Interview: Rescued!
• present perfect & simple past • emphasis with *it* & *what*	• personalizing* • brainstorming • choosing • making inferences • practicing • lateral thinking	• Lateral thinking: Meeting new people
• *when* & *if* clauses + modal *should/shouldn't* • relative clauses with *whose/who/who is*	• discovering* • selective listening • skimming • brainstorming • evaluating • cooperating	• Discussion: Caring and sharing
• passives: past & perfect forms • reported speech	• classifying* • selective listening • brainstorming • personalizing • making inferences • predicting	• Spot the difference: Wild party

* The asterisked Learning Strategies are explicitly taught in the unit. The others are used passively.

* The asterisked Learning Strategies are explicitly taught in the unit. The others are used passively.

Language Focus Structures	Learning Strategies	Communication Challenges
• review of past & perfect tenses • *supposed to*	• selective listening* • personalizing • cooperating • making inferences • skimming • self-evaluation	• Group task: Sequencing information
• complex passives • idioms	• cooperating* • selective listening • matching • personalizing • skimming • reflecting	• Debate: Graffiti
		• Group work: Evaluating others' opinions

* The asterisked Learning Strategy is explicitly taught in the unit. The others are used passively.

Atlas is a four-level ESL/EFL course for young adults and adults. Its learner-centered, task-based approach motivates learners and helps to create an active, communicative classroom.

Atlas represents an important step forward in language learning material. In **Atlas** topics, tasks, grammar, pronunciation, vocabulary, functions, notions, and learning-how-to-learn are all integrated. It is a complete teaching resource that can be used in a wide range of teaching situations. At the same time, it provides teachers with a unique opportunity to enhance and further develop their own classroom teaching skills.

Atlas can be used with existing curricula, courses, and methodologies. In addition, for those teachers who wish to explore new classroom approaches and techniques, this **Atlas** Teacher's Extended Edition offers a range of Optional activities and Variations on standard tasks, with explanations and comments.

Each book in the **Atlas** series is designed for a particular level of learner. Book 1 is for beginners, Book 2 is for high beginning learners or false beginners, Book 3 is for intermediate level learners, and Book 4 is for high intermediate learners. Each level of **Atlas** is designed to cover between 60–90 hours of classroom instruction.

In **Atlas**, students learn by using language creatively rather than by simply memorizing and reproducing it. Each unit is built on a task-based syllabus with a specific functional and grammatical focus and a relevant, contemporary, topical orientation. The topics, chosen to facilitate interesting and challenging communication, come from science and technology and popular culture as well as from everyday functional areas of communication.

This Book

Book 4 is for high intermediate learners. Some students may have already completed Book 3 before they begin Book 4. However, this is not necessary; high intermediate level students may begin with Book 4. Some of the themes and language points dealt with in Book 3 are reintroduced in more challenging ways in Book 4.

Course Components

Each level of this course consists of the following components:

- student's book
- teacher tape
- workbook
- workbook tape
- teacher's extended edition
- video
- assessment package

Approach

Atlas is unique in the following ways:

1. Atlas is learner-centered

Atlas focuses on helping learners to develop strategies that will help them learn. Developing strategies for learning a language is just as important as learning specific language items, and **Atlas** actively involves learners in the process of learning how to learn. It does this in a number of ways:

- goals and objectives are clearly explained to the learner;
- learners are involved in actively communicating with each other and with the teacher;
- as well as learning language, learners are taught about the learning process through a focus on learning strategies;
- learners are involved in making choices about their learning: choices about tasks, content, and the direction of the learning;
- learners are involved in monitoring their own progress;
- learners are encouraged to explore ways of learning that work for them;

- learners are given opportunities to predict, interpret, and make deductions from general to specific.

In addition, **Atlas** makes learning more meaningful by encouraging students to relate the material to their own knowledge and experience.

The following table shows the learning strategies that are presented in this course.

2. Atlas Uses a Task-Based Approach

Recent second language acquisition research shows that communicative interaction in the target language is very important for language

TASK TYPE	DEFINITION / EXAMPLE
CLASSIFYING	Putting things that are similar together in groups *Example: Study a list of proper names and classify them into male and female.*
PREDICTING	Predicting what is to come in the learning process *Example: Look at unit title and objectives and predict what will be learned.*
BRAINSTORMING	Thinking of as many new words and ideas as one can *Example: Work in a group and think of as many occupations as you can.*
SELECTIVE LISTENING	Listening for key words and information without trying to understand every word. *Example: Listen to a conversation and decide where the people are.*
PERSONALIZING	Learners share their own opinions, feelings, and ideas about a subject. *Example: Read a letter from a person in trouble, and say what you would do.*
SCANNING	Looking quickly through a written text for specific information *Example: Look at the text and decide if it is a newspaper article, a letter, or an advertisement.*
CONVERSATIONAL PATTERNS	Using expressions to start conversations and keep them going *Example: Match formulaic expressions to situations.*
COOPERATING	Sharing ideas and learning with other students *Example: Work in small groups to read a text and complete a table.*
DISCOVERING	Looking for patterns in language *Example: Study a conversation and discover the rule for forming the simple past tense.*
PRACTICING	Doing controlled exercises to improve knowledge and skills *Example: Listen to a conversation, and practice it with a partner.*
ROLE-PLAYING	Pretending to be somebody else and using the language for the situation you are in *Example: You are a reporter. Use the information from the reading to interview the writer.*

development. **Atlas** uses communication and learning tasks as the central building blocks in the curriculum, and the tasks are linked to the overall goals and objectives of the course.

Each unit contains two "task chains," in which succeeding tasks draw on and exploit the tasks that have come before. The advantage of task chains is that new learning builds on what learners already know. This is an essential element in successful learning. In **Atlas,** each new task gives learners the chance to practice language they have learned in earlier tasks and to build on and extend this.

3. Atlas Uses Authentic Data

Another important feature of the **Atlas** series is the use of authentic and simulated data. By "authentic data" we mean any language (spoken or written) that has not been specifically produced for the purposes of language instruction. We have included authentic and simulated texts because specially written texts and dialogues do not, by themselves, adequately prepare learners for the kinds of language they will meet outside the language learning situation. **Atlas** provides learners with opportunities to work with authentic texts. The simulated texts and dialogues have been developed with reference to authentic texts and genuine communicative contexts and reflect these as closely as possible.

4. Atlas Takes a Communicative Approach to Teaching Grammar and Discourse

Atlas takes an organic approach to grammar rather than a linear one. A linear view of language acquisition assumes that learners learn one thing perfectly, before moving to the next— i.e., the learner masters item a, then item b, then item c, and so on. **Atlas** presents a different view of language acquisition. We have followed recent second language acquisition research which shows that learners acquire a number of features all at once, imperfectly. Learning is organic rather than linear, and language grows in the same way as a flower grows, and not step by step in the way that a wall is built.

Because grammar is critical in developing communicative skills, **Atlas** introduces grammar tasks within real communication contexts. The grammar tasks are also designed to involve the learners in actively thinking about how English works. Learners are not given grammar rules to memorize and apply; they are invited instead to use the examples and models in the material to recognize language patterns, and work out language rules for themselves.

5. Book Organization

The book is divided into fifteen units, each organized around a particular topic or theme, for example, Unit 1: Celebrations, Unit 6: That's a Smart Idea, Unit 13: Time For a Change. Each unit includes a Warm-Up page with unit goals and introductory exercises, two Task Chains, two Language Focus pages, and a Self-Check page. Communication Challenge activities and grammar summaries for each unit are found at the back of the book. Units 5, 10, and 15 are review units that look back at the language covered in the previous four units.

6. General Teaching Strategies

Reading

Atlas presents a wide range of reading texts and includes tasks that involve different reading strategies.

Helping students to develop reading skills

Learners often feel that they must understand every word or their reading is not successful. This is not true. It is important to explain to students that there are many different ways of reading. How we read is determined by our purpose in reading. Sometimes we need to read texts very carefully and even slowly to make sure we have understood everything correctly. We read in detail like this when we read instructions for a new machine we want to use. But often we read just to get the main idea of the text, as in a magazine article or newspaper. This is called skimming. Or we read to find specific information and ignore the rest of the text. This is called scanning. We scan when we look up the TV program to find out what's on at 8 o'clock.

Atlas provides opportunities for students to skim and scan as well as to read for detailed information. In helping to develop reading strategies, you need to prepare them for what they are to read and why they are to read it. For example, are they to read for specific information? For details? For main ideas? They need to understand that the way we read something is determined by the kind of text it is—and by our purpose in reading it.

The goal of reading tasks is to help students understand some or all of the text. You can make comprehension easier for students if you prepare them for what they are going to read. Preparation tasks include brainstorming words and ideas linked to the text, discussing students' own experiences and knowledge, discussing possible contexts for the text, building up expectations of meaning, and so providing motivation to read. Learners are usually highly motivated to read each other's writing, and in **Atlas** there are many tasks where learners have the opportunity to do this.

Writing

Atlas presents a wide range of writing tasks that cover a variety of writing strategies.

Helping students to develop writing skills

Learners often feel stressed by writing tasks because they feel that they must write completely correct English at the first attempt. It is easier for students if the writing tasks are not individual tasks but are group or pair tasks, where two or more people work together to produce just one piece of writing. When the learners are producing their own written work, always allow time for them to write more than one draft. Let learners correct and revise, with your help, or by helping each other, so that the final draft is not the first draft. This enables students to learn from their own mistakes and relieves the pressure of producing a perfect piece of writing at the first attempt.

It is important to explain to students that, as with reading, there are many different ways of writing. How we write is determined by our reason for writing and by whom we are writing for. Sometimes we need to write rather formally, as in a business letter or job application, but often we write very informally or casually, as in notes, phone messages, or postcards, and this writing is much closer to spoken language.

You can make writing easier for students by always providing models of the kinds of texts you want the learners to produce. For example, if they are to write a postcard to a friend or a telephone message, or a business fax, show some examples of these, even if you have to produce these examples yourself. Talk about the features of the text, for example, whether the language is formal or friendly, or whether it has complete sentences or is abbreviated in places.

Listening

An important strategy in this course is selective listening. It is important to stress to students that, as with reading, it is not necessary to understand every word because at different times we listen in different ways and for different purposes. How we listen is determined by our reason for listening, by our knowledge of what we are listening to, and by what we are listening for. Sometimes we need to understand all, or almost all, of what we hear, but often we are only listening for part of what people are saying.

Helping students to develop listening skills   You can make listening easier for students if you prepare them for what they are going to hear. Prediction tasks are a very important part of developing listening skills. Such tasks involve class discussion about what students are going to hear. This may involve predicting the topic or even predicting what people will actually say. Prediction tasks give students the chance to engage in a free exchange of ideas and so to listen to each other, but they also prepare students for what they will listen to. When we listen for something in particular—for example, to verify our own prediction—this raises our level of concentration and improves overall listening comprehension.

Many classroom listening tasks involve listening to recordings or videos, and **Atlas** provides these important resources. But do not let students ignore the fact that listening skills can also be developed whenever students listen to you or to each other—in class discussions and in pair or group work.

Listening and repeating is important for pronunciation and for grammatical awareness. Many tasks in **Atlas** engage students in repeating and practicing what they have heard.

Speaking

The speaking tasks in **Atlas** focus on a number of different speaking skills—discussions, interviews, surveys, role-plays, as well as practice and repeating tasks.

Each of the following activities focuses on speaking skills.

Left Margin model sentences and conversations set off in special type have several purposes. They build confidence, they provide language models for some of the speaking tasks in the communication chains and challenges, and they give students an opportunity to improve their fluency and pronunciation.

Discussions   The purpose of discussion tasks is to give students opportunities to practice talking about their own experiences, not necessarily for them to agree or disagree with the text or with each other. You may decide to set a time limit of only a few minutes for a discussion or allow it to continue for as long as students are interested and actively involved.

Discussions can be of two kinds. They can be very open, aimed at giving students the chance to air their views freely and to gain more confidence in speaking English. The focus is on the content of the discussion, that is, saying what one thinks and why, and exchanging ideas with others. Or they can be more controlled, focusing not only on what students think and say but also on how they say it, that is, giving attention to the use of correct language, both grammar and pronunciation.

Where possible, discussion tasks of either kind should give students opportunities to extend their thinking beyond what is familiar and known, so that they become aware of other ways of looking at the issue beyond what they already know and believe.

Pair work

Pair work tasks are designed to give learners a chance to exchange ideas and information, to compare thoughts and feelings about the learning, and to learn from each other. It is important that learners experience this important part of classroom learning and not feel that they can only learn from the teacher. Cooperating or sharing ideas with other students means learning together and is an important learning strategy. Many pair work tasks involve interviewing other individuals in the class, or carrying out surveys. The survey is a valuable task for practicing speaking, but, when doing surveys, many students concentrate on gathering information and do a minimum of talking. To make this a useful speaking exercise, mingle with the students during the activity and ensure that they ask the questions **in full** and **from memory**. They can refer to their survey form before asking each question, but they should ask the question without reading. Make sure the survey question is asked and answered orally. Do not allow the students to simply read and/or write on each other's papers. And make sure that students use the correct question forms.

Group work

One of the advantages of group learning is the opportunities it provides for learners to communicate with each other. Like pair work, group work is a way of giving learners a chance to express their thoughts freely and discuss the learning. Group work can be more focused if students are asked to concentrate on a specific question or issue. If class discussions are done in small groups rather than as a whole class, more students have more opportunities to speak.

One important kind of group work is role-playing:

Role-plays involve pretending to be someone else and using language appropriate for a specific situation. Role-plays give opportunities for practicing language in a range of different contexts.

In all speaking tasks it is very important to give adequate time for learners to prepare for what they will have to say. Allow students time to practice the language structures or functions before they have to perform. Do not ask learners to use language before they have heard examples of what they are to say.

Class work

A number of the tasks in the course are designed as whole class activities. Brainstorming, often done as a whole class activity, is sharing as many thoughts and ideas as possible about a given topic. This is a good way for students to practice English, but it is also a good learning strategy because by hearing others' opinions, students can broaden their own views and learn about other ways of thinking.

Whole class activities make it possible to carry out more controlled discussion and are a most efficient way of giving all students information or instruction. Whole class activities are also particularly suitable for pre-task activities, to review previous learning, or to ascertain what learners already know.

Pronunciation

Pronunciation is an important part of communicative competence, and, like all language skills, it should be taught in context. Beyond a basic level, practicing discrete items of pronunciation such as minimal pair drill is not particularly effective for developing comprehensible pronunciation. However, it is important to provide students with contextualized pronunciation practice by focusing on pronunciation in the model dialogues that appear in most of the language focus sections of each unit. For these to be effective, it is important that you monitor and correct pronunciation, concentrating in particular on the stress, rhythm, and intonation.

Vocabulary

Increasing vocabulary is an important part of language learning, and each unit in **Atlas** has a section where vocabulary is reviewed and extended. It is important for students to realize that all language learning involves encountering new vocabulary and that there are a number of strategies they can use when they come across words that they do not know.

Helping students to develop vocabulary skills

There are some important ways that learners can use to check how well they know a word. Here is a useful checklist.

1. Can you recognize the word when you hear it—what it sounds like?
2. Can you recognize the word when you see it—the spelling, what it looks like? This includes being able to distinguish it from similar words.
3. Can you recall its meaning?
4. Do you know more than one meaning for the word?
5. Do you know shades of meaning for the word when you find it in different contexts?
6. Do you know the grammatical patterns the word most often occurs in?

7. Do you know the limitations on using the word, according to function and situation?
8. Do you know which words are commonly found together with the word in English—what words it will collocate with?

Encourage your students to:

1. use their knowledge of language and the world to figure out meanings.
2. use the situation or context to make intelligent guesses about the meaning of new words.
3. use their own life experiences to help them work out the meaning of text and individual words.
4. use syntactic, semantic, and contextual clues to help them work out meanings of unknown words in a text.
5. use visual and other non-linguistic clues.
6. use clues within words. Can they see other words or parts of a word within it? Prefix, suffix, root?
7. use information that has already gone before (in the conversation or in the text) to help construct meaning.
8. try to recall if they have heard/seen the word before. If so, where? In what context? Does it look like another word they know?
9. record vocabulary in a systematic way, a way that suits their own learning style and preferences.
10. use English-English dictionaries when possible rather than bilingual dictionaries.
11. use other learners and the teacher as a source of help.

Using dictionaries in class time should be avoided except when dealing with dictionary skills and strategies or where the task specifically requires it.

Review and Correction

There is a great deal of integration and recycling in the **Atlas** course. Learners have many opportunities to review and reprocess key language points in meaningful contexts. Many tasks allow for ongoing teacher correction while the students are working. Opportunities for teacher monitoring and correction are built into tasks in all the four skills—reading, writing, listening, and speaking. In addition, each unit has a self-checking section where learners can evaluate their progress, and there is a review unit after every four units.

Classroom management

Students learn in different ways, and to meet their different learning styles and strategies **Atlas** incorporates a range of different learning tasks, moving from individual work to pair and group work and back again from pair and group work to individual work to the whole class.

How Each Unit Is Organized

Unit Map

Unit Goals
Warm Up
Task Chain 1
Language Focus 1
Task Chain 2
Language Focus 2
Self-Check
Communication
   Challenge
Grammar Summary

Guidelines for Teaching a Unit

Unit Goals

The Unit Goals section gives teachers the chance to discuss learning goals with students. These goals provide learners with a sense of direction and progress in their learning. This is a very important part of learning, and the discussion at the beginning of each unit should include information about the topic and the kinds of tasks that students will work with in the unit. Each goal is followed by one or more sentences showing the goal in use.

Examples:

> In this unit, you will:
> **Exchange personal information**
> *"My name is Mike. What's your name?"*
> *"Where are you from?"*
> *"I'm from Tokyo."*
>
> **Describe yourself and other people**
> *"I'm twenty-three. I have dark hair."*
> *"Laura is fifty-five. She has green eyes."*
>
> **Introduce others**
> *"This is Yoko."*

You may choose to explain the grammar that students will practice in the unit.

Example:

> In this unit, you will:
> **Practice using the modal** *can*
> *"Can I smoke in here?"*
> *"Maria can speak five languages."*

You might also choose to talk about the kinds of texts that the students will work with in the unit. If you choose to do this, you should talk about both spoken and written texts.

Example:

> In this unit we will listen to friends talking together, read postcards from others, and write postcards to friends or family.
>
> In this unit you will listen to phone messages and read phone messages and faxes.

Warm-Up

The purpose of the warm-up section is to introduce students to some of the language patterns and vocabulary they will meet in the unit. It also provides an overview of the topics and content.

During the warm-up, and whenever possible in the unit, opportunities should be taken to relate the content of the unit to the students' own background knowledge and interests. This helps to motivate the students. Many warm-ups also contain model dialogues to provide students with initial fluency practice.

Task Chains

Each unit has two task chains, which are sequences of interrelated tasks. Some tasks in each unit are optional, and you may choose not to do them. The readings and listenings in the task chain present students with models of language and how it is used. Sometimes there are tasks where students have to use the language in the same way as it is used in the model.

In the task chains, new learning builds on what learners already know. This is an essential part of successful learning. In **Atlas** each new task gives learners the chance to practice language they have learned in earlier tasks and to build on their learning.

For example, in Unit 11, Task Chain 2, students are involved in exploring things that influ-

ence people's lives, especially in childhood, and cause them to make the decisions they do. The chain evolves through the following tasks:

> Task 1: Students create questions for the responses famous people have given about things that influenced them in their childhood. Students then discuss these with a partner.

> Task 2: Students listen to and discuss three conversations in which people talk about the things that influenced them, and led them to their current occupations.

> Task 3: Students read and discuss a magazine article which discusses, from a psychological perspective, the influences in childhood that are most significant in determining what kind of adults we become.

> Task 4: Students write and discuss the three most influential people, places and events in their own lives, to this point, and why they have been so important.

Some tasks in each unit are **optional.** These are an element added to the primary task, and you may choose not to do them if, for example, there is not time for more work at this point or if the task required learners to supply information or create language that has not been specifically dealt with in the unit.

There are also **Variation** tasks in each unit. These are alternative ways of doing the primary task; that is, you do the Variation task rather than the task as it is set out in the Student book. Teachers may choose not to do the Variation task, but those who do will need to explain to learners that this task is an alternate way of doing the learning activity and replaces the task in their book.

Variation tasks give teachers who wish to try new approaches or new teaching techniques a chance to do so and at the same time relate the new approach to the tasks in the student book, which represent techniques and methods that are more familiar.

You Choose

An important learning-how-to-learn feature in this course is teaching students to make choices. "You choose" gives opportunities for students to choose by presenting more than one task and having students select which of the tasks they want to do. At first these can be done as a whole class exercise until students become familiar with the concept and the practice of choosing for themselves.

Language Focus

The language focus sections analyze specific grammatical and functional points that have been presented in the preceding task chain, and include practice tasks for using the language in context. These sections allow you to strike a healthy balance between attention to form and function in language on the one hand and learner-centered communicative activities on the other.

Most language focus sections begin with a short dialogue or reading that reviews the language covered in the task chain. This allows students to refamiliarize themselves with the language to be practiced. Following the language model are several activities that range from controlled, cloze-type exercises to open-ended communicative tasks. You can choose to do the tasks in a different order than they are in the book. You may also omit exercises that you feel are not appropriate for your students.

The reason for placing each language focus after each task chain is that in this way learners are made familiar with the language in use before they begin to analyze it in detail and before they are required to use it themselves.

Alternative

Teachers sometimes prefer to present grammar before moving on to communicative tasks. This is a perfectly appropriate alternative. Or you may choose, just in certain units, to do the language focus work before involving learners in the communicative task chains.

Do You Know the Rule?

Occasionally you will find in this section a feature called "DO YOU KNOW THE RULE?" This feature is designed to help students to identify patterns in language and use these to figure out for themselves a language pattern or rule. Recognizing patterns and inducing rules is a more effective way of learning than simply memorizing rules.

Self-Check

The self-check sections are an important and integral part of the course. In this section learners are invited to review the unit. Self-monitoring and self-reflection are important aspects of learning how to learn and also help students to evaluate their progress.

Students first write down new words and structures they have learned. Some of these tasks can be done out of class and brought to the next lesson. If possible, students should do these tasks without looking back at the unit. Students then evaluate their progress. The self-evaluation tasks also serve to remind students of the goals of the unit. Finally, students are invited to reflect on ways in which they can improve their learning skills. They are helped in this by sample statements from other learners. As students progress through the book, the Self-Check becomes their own personalized learning journal.

Communication Challenge

At the end of each unit there is a reference to the unit's Communication Challenge with the page number(s) on which it will be found. The purpose of the Communication Challenge is to provide the learners with an opportunity to reinforce and practice language they have learned in the task chains. The Communication Challenge may be an information gap, a role-play, a guided discussion, or a problem-solving task.

Grammar Summaries

The grammar summaries, on pages 129 through 134, provide, for each unit, a quick review of the grammar taught in the unit. Consistent with the inductive approach to grammar in **Atlas,** they present examples, not rules, for the structures dealt with in the Language Focus sections of the unit. These can be especially valuable as reminders of what was taught in the unit and for additional practice. Call attention to them when you introduce the book to the students and when you assign the Self-Check pages at the end of each unit.

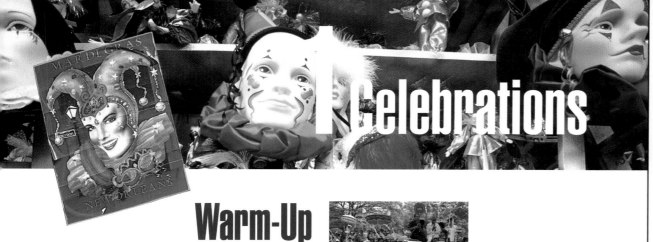

Celebrations

Warm-Up

Unit Goals

In this unit you will:

Give details about special events

"The festival will start in the morning."

Make and respond to invitations and requests

"We would be delighted if you could make it to our wedding."

"In my country, people always give gifts for birthdays, weddings, and the birth of a child. And they sometimes bring small gifts, such as flowers or chocolates, when they go to a dinner party."

Thailand

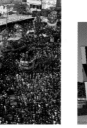

Brazil

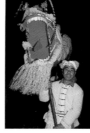

Australia

Hong Kong

1 Group Work Discussion. What do you think the people are celebrating?

2 a Make a list of the things you celebrate and put them into the following categories.

Personal
(*things you, your family, and friends celebrate*)
- your parents' wedding anniversary
- your birthday

....

....

Public
(*things other people also celebrate*)
- the last day of school

- New Year's Eve

....

....

b Compare your list with another student.

3 Group Work In this unit we will look at the custom of giving gifts. When do people give gifts in your country?

📖 Student text page 9

Warm-Up

This section provides a context for the unit. It presents the language of giving details about special events and making and responding to invitations and requests.

Unit Goals. Read out each goal and sample language. Ask students to circle those they can do in English. Ask a representative number of students for their responses. This way, you can get an idea of the range in the group.

1. Ask students for their responses. Point out that celebrations are often very specific to one country or region.

2. (**a**) Mention to students that personal celebrations can vary greatly from individual to individual and family to family.

(**b**) Have each student trade lists with another student and compare responses.

3. Have students think about the occasions when people exchange gifts in their country. Then, in groups of three, they use the model language to discuss these customs. **Variation.** If students are all from the same country, region, or culture, have volunteers talk about gift-giving customs in families or in some other culture they know about or have lived in.

Task Chain 1: Festivals

Task 1. **(a)** With the whole class, brainstorm the kinds of celebrations that occur in different societies. List these on the board. Students can work in pairs or small groups.

(b) In pairs or small groups, students look at the pictures and match the festival with the place where it happens.
(Answers: Thailand—Water Festival; Brazil—Carnival; Australia—Festival of Arts; Hong Kong—Dragon Boat Festival)

Task 2. **(a)** 🎧 Students listen individually and number the segments as they hear them.
(Answers: 2, 3, 1, 4)

(b) 🎧 Students listen again and circle any places/festivals from Task 1b that they hear.
(Answers: Places—Australia, Hong Kong; Festivals—Festival of Arts, Carnival, Water Festival, Dragon Boat Festival)

(c) 🎧 Students fill in the chart after listening to the tape for a third time. **Variation.** Have students work in pairs to fill in the chart.
(Answers: Jack—Australia, Festival of Arts: music, art, literature, theater; Paula—Brazil, Carnival: nonstop music and dancing; Suriwong—Thailand, Water Festival: religious festival, people drenched with water; Nina—Hong Kong, Dragon Boat Festival: religious festival but very enjoyable)

Learning Strategy. In each unit, students practice different learning strategies. Here, they are given instruction and practice on one particular reading strategy—scanning.

Task 3. Working individually, students compare the information in the letter with the information in the brochure. Have them underline the parts of the letter that are incorrect. Then have them rewrite the letter to correct the information.

(Continued on page 11.)

Task Chain 1 Festivals

Celebrations

religious

Task 1

a **Group Work** Brainstorm. What types of celebrations do societies have? Make a list.

b Look at the pictures on page 9 and draw lines to match the places with their festivals.

Place	Festival
1 Thailand	Dragon Boat Festival
2 Brazil	Water Festival
3 Australia	Carnival
4 Hong Kong	Festival of Arts

Task 2

a 🎧 Listen to the tape. Number the following segments (1 to 4) when you hear them.

.... casual conversation
.... tour guide
.... TV talk show
.... advertisement

b 🎧 Listen again. Look at Task 1b, and circle the names of the places and festivals that you hear.

c 🎧 Listen once more. Which festivals are these people talking about? What do they say about the festivals? Fill in the chart.

NAME	PLACE	FESTIVAL	TYPE/CHARACTERISTICS
Jack			
Paula			
Suriwong			
Nina			

LEARNING STRATEGY

Scanning = searching a text for specific information

Task 3

The writer of the following letter has gotten some of his facts wrong. Scan the brochure and then correct the letter for him.

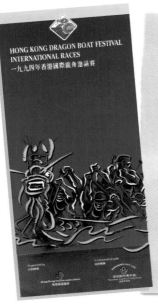

Dragon Boat Festival

The 2,000-year-old Dragon Boat (*Tuan Ng*) Festival commemorates the death in the third century B.C. of Chinese national hero Qu Yuan. Qu Yuan drowned himself in the Mi Lo River to protest the corrupt government. Legend has it that villagers raced their boats towards him in a vain attempt to save his life, striking their paddles on the water, beating drums, and throwing rice dumplings wrapped in bamboo leaves into the river. The paddles and drums were supposed to scare the fish away and stop them from eating Qu Yuan's body.

Today rice dumplings wrapped in bamboo leaves are a traditional festival food, but the real highlight of the festival is the colorful Dragon Boat races. The special boats, which range in length from 38 to 120 feet, have ornately carved and painted dragon heads and tails. Each boat carries a crew of 22 or more paddlers.

Race participants train in earnest for the competition. Sitting two abreast with a steersman at the back and a drummer at the front, the paddlers race to reach the finishing line, urged on by the pounding drums and the roar of the crowd.

The Hong Kong Dragon Boat Festival and International Races take place on a Saturday and Sunday in the middle of June. One hundred and sixty teams (including 32 from overseas) enter the races, which are held off the Tsim Sha Tsui East waterfront.

Dear Sergio,

I've just had the greatest time in Hong Kong at the Dragon Boat Festival, which is held here every June. The festival has been going on for 1,500 years. It's meant to celebrate Chinese Emperor Qu Yuan who drowned while swimming in the Mi Lo River. Apparently some sailors tried to rescue him, but failed. They hit the water with their paddles, beat drums, and threw rice dumplings wrapped in bamboo leaves into the river for him to eat. The races held these days are based on this event that was supposed to have happened all those years ago. There are people and boat racing teams here from twenty different countries. It was a fantastic event, and one that I can thoroughly recommend. I'll write again soon. Next week I'm off to Bangkok.

Sincerely,
Joshua

Task 4

You choose. Do **A** or **B**.

A **Group Work** Think of a festival or special event and describe what you do on that day. Your classmates will guess what festival or event it is.

B Think of the most interesting or exciting holiday you've ever had and describe it to your classmates.

(Answers: The following corrections should be made—1,500 years should be 2,000 years; Qu Yuan was not an emperor; villagers, not sailors, tried to save him; the rice dumplings were not for Qu Yuan to eat; the races commemorate the event but are not based on it; thirty-three, not twenty, countries are represented.)

Task 4.   It is very important to link new learning to the learner's own experiences. In this task students talk about events they have experienced and know well. Those who choose **A** work in groups and try to guess the festival from the description. This task will work best if the students are all familiar with the festival's events. It may not work so well if students are from different countries, or from very different cultures within the same country, and are not familiar with the festivals or events that might be described. Those who choose **B** should prepare a descriptive narrative no longer than two minutes. Have them consider different aspects of the holiday—weather, activities, food, company, traveling there and back.

Language Focus 1: Prepositional phrases

1. (a) Have students read the article individually and correct any mistakes they find. Check answers with the whole class.
(Answers: in Deep Springs, for five years, on the first day of Fall, at night, on foot, to other destinations)

(b) In pairs, students read the article again and mark any other prepositional phrases. Check answers with the whole class.
(Answers: near the edge of town; in music, art, and even theater; to the festival; from all over the world; for the festival)

2. Working individually, students put the prepositions into the appropriate columns. Circulate and provide assistance where necessary.
(Answers: Place—in, under, to, on, into, above, onto, over, towards; Time—in, since, during, for, over)

3. (a) Working individually, students read through the sentences and then fill in the missing prepositions.
(Answers: 1. In, at, until; 2. after; 3. under *or* in; 4. since; 5. into. Note: possible speakers will vary.)

(b) In small groups, students compare and discuss their responses and decide whose are the most interesting and original.

4. Give pairs of students time to read and think about information they might write about themselves, using the phrases in the list and the model language as a guide. This task could be done as a written exercise or as a speaking task. Circulate and check grammar, spelling, and pronunciation.
(Answers will vary.)

Language Focus 1 Prepositional phrases

1 a Correct the mistakes in the underlined phrases.

b Pair Work Can you find any other prepositional phrases? Underline them.

> I lived <u>on Deep Springs</u> <u>during five years</u> and found it really interesting. Each year, there was an arts and crafts festival, beginning <u>in the first day of Fall.</u> The festival was held in an old factory near the edge of town. It was great, because the organizers catered to many different tastes in music, art, and even theater. While there were events during the day, the best performances were <u>in night.</u> People would come to the festival from all over the world. It used to get so crowded that we'd go there <u>in foot</u>, rather than in a car. People traveling through Deep Springs on their way <u>at other destinations</u> would often stop for the festival instead of going on to their intended destination.

PLACE	TIME	EITHER

2 Classify these prepositions according to whether they introduce phrases of place or time.

in	under	on	above	during	over
since	to	into	onto	for	towards

3 a Fill in the blanks with the correct prepositions. Now decide who you think might have made each statement.

Example: During the day I lie in bed, and then ...*at*... night I go out to work. *a security guard*

1. .... the morning, I get up .... five o'clock, and exercise .... about eight. ....

2. They ran .... me calling me terrible names. ....

3. We were .... the shelter of some trees when the lightning struck. ....

4. I haven't been back there .... they threw me out. ....

5. They've turned the place where I was born .... a tourist attraction. ....

b Group Work Compare responses. Who had the most interesting/original choices?

"Nothing much ever happens in the place where I was born, which is why I don't live there any more."

4 Pair Work Use these phrases to make statements that are true for you.

a in the morning
b for most of my childhood
c in the place where I was born
d during the summer
e since I was a young kid

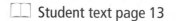

Task Chain 2 Gifts

"I'd give the tie to my brother for his birthday because it's loud and tasteless—just like him!"

Task 1

a Pair Work Discuss with a partner who you would give these gifts to and for what occasion.

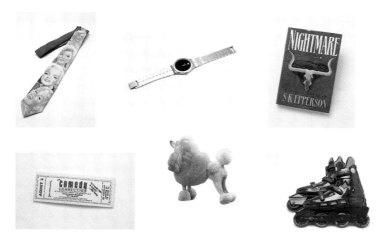

b Group Work Compare your choices with another pair's.

Task 2

a 🎧 Listen to the first interview and ask the teacher to stop the tape whenever you hear a question. Write the questions below.

....
....
....

b 🎧 Listen again and fill in the chart for all three interviews.

PERSON	FAVORITE GIFT	NEXT BIRTHDAY	OTHER PEOPLE	COST
Mariel				
Natasha				
Rod				

"Well, Natasha is most like me, because she chooses things that people wouldn't buy for themselves—just like me."

c Rank the people from most to least like you in terms of their gift-giving habits (1 to 3).

d Group Work Talk about your choices.

📖 Student text page 13

Task Chain 2: Gifts

Task 1. With the whole class, discuss the gifts in the picture, choosing at least two adjectives to describe each one. List these on the board.

(**a**) In pairs, students discuss who they would give each gift to and why. Make sure this is a speaking practice task and that students use the sample language as a guide.

(**b**) Combine pairs to discuss their choices.

Task 2. (**a**) 🎧 Play the tape and have students raise their hands at the point where they hear a question. Stop the tape at this point. Students write the question they have heard. **Optional.** At the end of the tape, have students work in pairs to compare their questions and correct them if they wish.
(Answers: any three of the four questions posed by the interviewer)

(**b**) 🎧 Play the tape again and have students work individually to complete the table.
(Answers: Mariel—baby doll, none, gives parties instead of gifts, high; Natasha—Italian cruise, year's supply of massages, something that reminds her of the other person, low; Rod—anything except socks and underwear, a fun-filled year, what the other person wants, whatever it takes)

(**c**) Still working individually, students think about which of the people have gift-giving habits similar to their own, and rank them.

(**d**) In small groups and using the model language as a guide, students compare and discuss their rankings.

Celebrations **13**

Celebrations **13**

Task 3. Give students time individually to read and answer the survey questions for themselves. Remind students of the dual purpose of surveys: to gather information and to practice speaking. Encourage students to memorize the questions so that when they are doing the survey they can ask them without reading. Have them record their survey responses on a separate sheet of paper. Call on students at random from around the class to give one or two answers from their survey.

Task 4. In pairs, students read the excerpts from the letters and notes, and match them to their writers. Circulate and provide assistance if necessary. Combine two or three pairs to compare and discuss their choices.
(Answers: surprise party—b; birthday party for elderly relative—d; inviting friend to party—a; wedding—c)

Task 5. (a) Give each student time to think about the birthday party. Students can choose an imaginary party or a party from their own experience.
Variation. Have students prepare their thoughts about this task before they come to the lesson.
   (b) In pairs, students compare and discuss their responses.

Task 3

Group Work Interview two classmates and fill in the chart.

	PERSON 1	PERSON 2
What's the nicest gift that you've received?		
What gift would you most like to receive?		
When do you give gifts?		
How do you choose gifts for others?		
How much do you usually spend?		

Task 4

Pair Work Study the following excerpts from letters and notes. Match each excerpt with its writer.

.... someone planning a surprise party for a friend
.... someone planning a birthday dinner for an elderly relative
.... someone inviting a friend to a party
.... someone inviting a relative to a wedding

a "I hope you can make it."

b "and most of the arrangements have been made. Unfortunately, I haven't been able to contact Mack. Do you think you'll see him at the game on Saturday? Remind him not to say a word, of course."

c "It will only be a small gathering, but John and I would be delighted if you could make it. The ceremony will be in the park, and then we'll go to John's parent's place for the reception."

d "We won't be able to eat too late, of course, but it would be great if you could make it."

Task 5

a Someone invites you to a birthday party, but you don't want to go. What are you most likely to do? Rank these options from most to least likely (1 to 5 or 6).

.... change the topic
.... say you are already busy
.... end the conversation without saying "yes" or "no."
.... remain silent
.... say you don't want to go
.... other (specify): ....

b **Pair Work** Compare your choices with another student's.

Language Focus 2 Modals: can/could/would/would mind

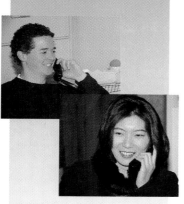

1 🎧 **Pair Work** Listen. Then practice the conversation.

A: Hello, Tomoko?
B: Oh, hi Jim.
A: I'm calling to see if you can come to my party on Saturday night.
B: I can't, sorry. I'm having dinner with a friend.
A: Would you be able to come later?
B: Well, I guess I could come around eleven. Would you mind if I brought my friend?
A: No, not at all. See you then.

2 a **Pair Work** Have a conversation, using these functions.

A: (Call up your partner.)
B: (Answer the phone.)
A: (Invite your friend to a birthday party/dinner/the movies.)
B: (Say no and give an excuse.)
A: (Suggest an alternative.)
B: (Accept or decline the alternative.)

b **Pair Work** Now change roles and have the conversation again.

3 Rank these requests from least formal to most formal (1 to 4).

.... I wonder if you'd mind copying this report for me?
.... Could you invite Mike to the party?
.... Would you mind if I brought Marco to your party?
.... Can you pass the ketchup?

4 a Which of these phrases would you use for the following situations?

1 "I wonder if you'd mind"
2 "Could you"
3 "Would you mind"
4 "Can you"

.... You want your younger brother/sister to hand you a book.
.... You want your teacher to tell you your exam results.
.... You want your best friend to pick up the tickets for a show.
.... You want a friend to write down a phone number for you.
.... You want a stranger to tell you the time.

b **Pair Work** Compare your responses with another student's response.

c **Pair Work** Take turns role playing these situations.

Language Focus 2: Modals:
can/could/would/would mind

1. 🎧 Play the tape. Remind students that the purpose of these conversations is to provide speaking practice. With this in mind, encourage students to try to say the lines from memory rather than simply reading them.

2. **(a)** With the whole class, read through the stages of the conversation. Have pairs of students decide on the information they will include in their two versions of the conversation. What kind of invitation is it? When? What excuse will each Speaker B give? What alternative will each Speaker A suggest? Will Speaker B accept or decline the alternative in each case? Then have the pairs decide on the exact language they will use in the conversation. They may make written notes if they wish, but do not allow them to write out the conversation in full. When they practice the conversation, they should refer to their notes as little as possible.

(b) Students swap roles and practice the conversation again.

3. Discuss with the whole class the concept of formal and informal language. Remind them that English is much less formal than many other languages. (Answers: 1. Can you; 2. Could you; 3. Would you mind if; 4. I wonder if you'd mind)

4. **(a)** Remind students that the level of politeness or formality required in these situations could vary in different cultures, in different communities, and even in different families. With the whole class, discuss and complete one example from the list. Then have students work individually to complete the others. (Answers will vary, but should follow the general sequence indicated in **3** above.)

(b) In pairs, students compare and discuss their responses.

(c) Still in pairs, students role-play each of the situations. Circulate and correct grammar and pronunciation as needed.

Self-Check

Communication Challenge

The Communication Challenge tasks provide opportunities for students to use, in a freer context, the language they have been learning. Challenge 1 is on page 111 of the student text, and suggestions for its use are on that page in this Teacher's Extended Edition.

1, 2, 3. Encourage students to complete the first three tasks without looking back at the unit.

4. (a) Have students write down responses. **Variation.** Have students choose three different people for the second sentence: someone they know very well, someone they know a little, and someone they have just met. Students should adjust their language to suit each context.
(b) Students work in small groups to brainstorm occasions to use the suggested language.

• Tell the class that summaries of the grammar points covered in each unit can be found at the back of their texts. The summary for Unit 1 is on page 129.

5. It is most important that learners develop skills and strategies for learning on their own. As much as possible, have students do tasks such as this one out of class and then discuss their responses with the whole class.

6. Have students work individually to check off the words that they know.

Self-Check

COMMUNICATION CHALLENGE

Pair Work Look at Challenge 1 on page 111.

1 Write down five new words you learned in this unit.

2 Write sentences using three of these new words.

3 Write three new sentences or questions you learned.

4 a

WHAT WOULD YOU SAY?

Your best friend invites you to his/her birthday party, but you can't make it.

You say:

You want someone to get you a book from the library.

You say:

You are telling friends about a festival you went to.

You say:

b Group Work Brainstorm ways to practice this language out of class. Imagine you are visiting an English-speaking country. Where/When might you need this language?

5 Out of Class Find out about a festival in your country. See if you can find out some unusual facts about the event. Bring the information to class and be prepared to talk about it.

6 Vocabulary check. Check [√] the words you know.

Adjectives/Adverbs			Nouns		Verbs		Prepositions
□ always	□ interesting	□ unfortunately	□ advertisement	□ gift	□ celebrate	□ remain	□ above
□ busy	□ loud	□ usually	□ alternative	□ habit	□ choose	□ rescue	□ during
□ casual	□ personal	□ vain	□ celebration	□ hero	□ commemorate	□ respond	□ for
□ colorful	□ public		□ ceremony	□ invitation	□ drown	□ scan	□ in
□ corrupt	□ silent		□ competition	□ news broadcast	□ get up		□ into
□ delighted	□ sometimes		□ conversation	□ participant	□ invite	**Modal Verbs**	□ on
□ elderly	□ special		□ custom	□ program	□ lend	□ can	□ onto
□ exciting	□ sports		□ details	□ reception	□ practice	□ could	□ over
□ fantastic	□ tasteless		□ excuse	□ request	□ protest	□ would	□ since
□ gift-giving	□ traditional		□ festival	□ talk show	□ race	□ would mind	□ to
							□ towards

2 Believe It or Not

Unit Goals

In this unit you will:

Express degrees of belief and disbelief

"I find that hard to believe."

Give details about events

"The place where the ship went down was just off the coast."

Warm-Up

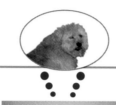
Picture 1

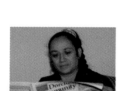
Picture 2

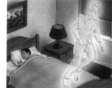
Picture 3

Picture 4

1 a Match the pictures with the statements in Task 1b. Write the number of the picture in the blank at the left.

b How believable do you find these statements? Circle a number.

PICTURE NUMBER	STATEMENT	COMPLETELY BELIEVABLE				COMPLETELY UNBELIEVABLE
....	"My brother and I can tell what each other is thinking—we are telepathic."	1	2	3	4	5
....	"I saw a ghost last year."	1	2	3	4	5
....	"I once experienced astral travel—I actually left my body for several minutes."	1	2	3	4	5
....	"The horoscope in the newspaper last week predicted everything that happened to me this week."	1	2	3	4	5

2 **Group Work** Compare your responses with three or four other students.

📖 Student text page 17

Warm-Up

Unit Goals.   This unit presents the language of expressing degrees of belief and disbelief, and giving details about events. Read out each goal and sample language. Ask students to circle those they can do in English. Ask a number of students for their responses. This way, you can get an idea of the range in the group.

1. **(a)** Working individually, students look at the pictures, read the statements, and then match them. (Answers: "My brother"—4; "I saw a ghost"—1; "I once experienced astral travel"—3; "The horoscope"—2)

(b) Students read the statements again and decide how believable they think each statement is. They mark their opinion of the statement on the scale from 1, "Completely Believable," to 5, "Completely Unbelievable."

2. In groups of four or five, students compare and discuss their responses. Pick four students at random to give their opinions to the class. Then ask for four other students with very different opinions from the first four.

Task Chain 1: Stranger than fiction

Task 1. **(a)** Working individually, students mark the words that they already know. **Variation.** Have students discuss the words and put them into groups or categories—for example, adjectives, nouns, verbs, or words with the same number of syllables.

(b) In small groups, and using the sample language, students talk about the words in the list that they know well and any words that are new or unfamiliar to them. **Variation.** Have students create a story using as many of the words from the list as possible. This can be either a spoken or a written task.

Task 2. **(a)** ∩ This is a selective listening task. Play the tape, and have students listen first for the two events and then write them down. Then play the tape a second time, and ask students to listen for what is unusual about the two events.
(Answers: 1—intuition about harm to neighbor; apparent telepathy. 2—two people being able to think of same number most of the time; highly improbable)

(b) ∩ In pairs, students compare and discuss their responses. Play the tape again so that students can confirm their answers.

(c) ∩ Play the tape once again. Have students indicate whether they believe in telepathy or not. This can be a free discussion, with the emphasis more on exchanging ideas and opinions than on accuracy.
(Answers: Pete—believes; Mark—doesn't believe; Gina—not sure)

Task 3. **(a)** Remind students of the reading strategy of skimming—i.e., reading quickly to see what the article is about, not reading carefully for details.
(Answer: telepathy)

Task Chain 1 Stranger than fiction

Task 1

a Check [√] the words you know.

☐ weird	☐ happen	☐ relaxing
☐ junk food	☐ strange	☐ wrong
☐ uncomfortable	☐ ignore	☐ elderly
☐ compulsion	☐ lying	☐ knocked
☐ telepathy	☐ thoughts	☐ mental
☐ messages	☐ rubbish	☐ concentrate
☐ travel	☐ crazy	

"For me, the least familiar words are *compulsion* and *concentrate*. The most familiar are *messages* and *travel.*"

b **Group Work** Discussion. Which are the most familiar and least familiar words in the list?

Task 2

a ∩ Listen to the conversation. You will hear about two unusual events. What are the events? Why are they unusual?

EVENT	WHY IS IT UNUSUAL?
1	
2	

b ∩ Compare your responses with another student's responses and then listen again to check your answers.

c ∩ Listen once more. Who believes in telepathy, doesn't believe, isn't sure? Put a check [√] in the correct column.

	Believes	Not sure	Doesn't believe
Pete	☐	☐	☐
Mark	☐	☐	☐
Gina	☐	☐	☐

Task 3

a Skim the following story. What do you think it is about? Check [√] one box.

☐ telepathy   ☐ astral travel   ☐ coincidence

Lucien felt that Joan and Bill had an understanding on some deep level that people rarely achieve, something on a <u>psychic level</u> that you could actually feel. Sitting in the living room of their small apartment, he watched them play their favorite game. They sat at opposite ends of the room, and each one took a sheet of paper and divided it into nine squares, and drew a picture in each of the squares, and when they had finished they compared the drawings and there was an <u>uncanny correlation</u>—they had both drawn a scorpion, and they had both drawn a bottle, and they had both drawn a dog. About half the drawings were the same. To Lucien, the degree of telepathic communication was <u>spooky</u>.

From *Literary Outlaw: The Life and Times of William S. Burroughs*, by T. Morgan.

b Scan the story and decide which of the underlined words and phrases mean:

mysterious and a little frightening ....

extraordinary similarity ....

spiritual dimension ....

c Do you think that the story is unusual? Do you think that the event could simply have been a coincidence?

Task 4

a **Pair Work** Think of a number between 1 and 10. Write it on a piece of paper, but don't let your partner see. Concentrate on the number for ten seconds. Your partner will try to guess the number and write it on a piece of paper. Compare numbers. Repeat this several times. How often were you successful?

b **Pair Work** Now change roles and do the task again.

c **Group Work** Compare results with other class members.

Task 5

Group Work Discussion.

a Have you ever had an unusual experience similar to those discussed in Task 2?

b Do you know anybody else who has had experiences like these?

c Can you think of explanations other than telepathy to account for the events?

Student text page 19

(b) Remind students that there are different ways of reading. One reading strategy is scanning—that is, not reading carefully for every detail, but reading to find only specific information. Have students scan the article for the meaning of the underlined words and phrases.
(Answers: mysterious and a little frightening—spooky; extraordinary similarity—uncanny correlation; spiritual dimension—psychic level)
(c) Linking the learning to students' own life experiences and ideas is an important part of successful learning. Discuss the two questions with the whole class. Encourage students to give their own opinions regardless of what others think.

Task 4. (a, b) This is an enjoyable way to experiment with the idea of telepathy. Pairs of students try to see if they can influence the number their partner chooses just by thinking about it. Then have students swap roles and repeat the task.

(c) Ask one person from each pair to give the results of their experiment to the whole class—that is, how many times the partners thought of the same number. **Variation.** With the whole class, discuss whether students think that the results are due to telepathy or coincidence.

Task 5. (a, b, c) With the whole class, listen again to the conversations in Task 2. Then read each of the discussion questions and make sure everyone understands them. Have students work in small groups to discuss each question. Call on volunteers to relate to the whole class any interesting or unusual responses.

Language Focus 1: Short responses

1.   Read the questions through with the whole class to make sure that everyone understands them. Then have students work in pairs to match the questions and responses.
(Answers: a—Not since it said I'd win a million dollars; b—I find that hard to believe; c—No, not yet)

2.   (a) All students bring their own knowledge and attitudes to the learning. New learning will be successful only if it is personally relevant and meaningful. The most important way of making learning meaningful is to link it with what students already know and think. Have students work individually to read the questions and choose the response they would give. Make sure they understand that there is no right or wrong answer; this is simply a chance for them to express their own opinion. Elicit responses at random from around the class.
      (b) Have students work in pairs to practice asking and answering the questions. Students should give their responses from memory, without reading them. Make sure that all students practice both asking and answering.

3.   (a) Before students begin this task, brainstorm possible topics for the questions—for example, strange or unusual happenings. Then have students work individually to choose one or more of the topics and write questions or statements about them. Ask volunteers to give one or more responses.
      (b) In pairs, students practice the short exchanges, from memory if possible.

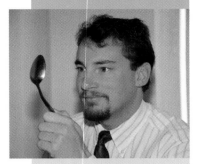

1 Pair Work Match the questions and responses and then practice them with your partner.

Questions

a Are you still reading that awful horoscope column in the newspaper?

b Did you know that I saw a ghost once when I was a kid?

c Have you seen the guy on TV who can bend spoons by looking at them?

Responses

.... I find that hard to believe.

.... No, not yet.

.... Not since it said I'd win a million dollars.

2 a Underline the response that you would give to these questions.

   1 Do you believe in telepathy?
      a) I used to.
      b) Not since I was a child.
      c) No, it's all in your head.

   2 Have you ever seen a ghost?
      a) Only once.
      b) No, not yet.
      c) No, but I expect to soon.

   3 Are you still practicing telepathy?
      a) Only occasionally.
      b) I never did.
      c) Not recently.

   4 Are you superstitious?
      a) Only occasionally.
      b) Yes, every time I see my former teacher.
      c) Not unless I'm waiting for my exam results.

   b Pair Work Now practice the questions and responses with a partner.

3 a Think of questions or statements for these responses.

   1 ....
      I find that hard to believe.
   2 ....
      You're kidding.
   3 ....
      Only on the weekend.
   4 ....
      No, not yet.

   b Pair Work Now practice them with a partner.

Task Chain 2 At least it's news!

Task 1

a **Group Work** Put these pictures in order to make a story.

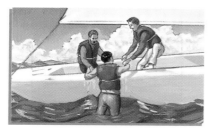

Picture ....

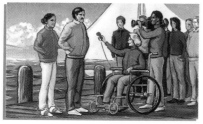

Picture ....

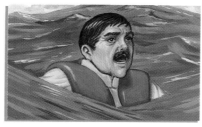

Picture ....

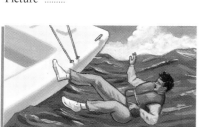

Picture ....

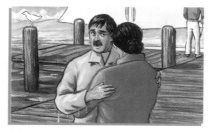

Picture ....

b Now tell the story using some of these words.

fell overboard	survived
rough conditions	pulled from water
taken ashore	reunited with wife

Task Chain 2: At least it's news!

Task 1. (a) This task allows students to compare their own perspectives with those of others in the class. One important aspect of classroom learning is this opportunity for students to see how others perceive and understand, and what strategies they use in learning. Have students work in groups to put the pictures into a sequence so they tell a story. Students will need to discuss and negotiate to arrive at a consensus.

(b) With the whole class, go through the list of terms. Make sure everyone understands them. Have students work in the same groups and tell their picture story by using as many of the terms from the list as possible. Give the groups at least five minutes to work on their story before asking them to tell it, but encourage them to create the story orally, *not* in writing.

Learning Strategy. This unit concentrates on predicting. Point out to your students that successful reading involves prediction, or trying to determine what might logically follow.

Task 2. (a) Before students read the article, remind them that opinions are often shared by many people, but this alone does not make them facts. This task concentrates on scanning. Have students read the article to find two facts and one opinion. Limit the reading to five minutes.
(Answers may vary. Sample answers: Facts—Estrada came ashore yesterday. He survived freezing conditions after falling overboard from his yacht. Opinion—Estrada is lucky to be alive.)

(b) In groups, students compare and discuss their responses. Make sure that they give reasons for their choices. The group may not arrive at consensus, but giving and supporting opinions is an important conversation skill, and this task gives students the chance to practice it.

(c) 🎧 Understanding language means being able to understand different codes. Recognizing and matching the same information in different codes is a valuable learning activity. Give students time to reread the newspaper report, and then play the tape. Individually, students fill in the chart, noting the similarities and differences between the two reports.
(Answers: For both similarities and differences, various answers are possible. Make sure that students can back up their responses with facts from the broadcast and the news report.)

(d) Ask for volunteers who can offer possible reasons that the two reports would differ.
(Answers will vary.)

Task 3. (a) It is important to give learners opportunities to share their personal experiences. Give students at least five minutes to think of some personal experiences and then choose one to tell to the group.
Variation. Have students choose the experience they will talk about before they come to the lesson.

(b) Have group members decide which experience was the most dramatic or interesting. Remind them that the objective of the discussion is to share ideas and opinions, not to arrive at consensus.

(c) Have one member of each group tell his or her story to the whole class.

Task 2

a Read the following newspaper story and see if you can find two facts and one opinion. Underline the facts and circle the opinion.

HEADLINE:

....

by Rebecca Hill

Champion yachtsman Pete Estrada came ashore at San Diego yesterday after being rescued from a harrowing five hours in the open ocean. Supposedly one of the best sailors in the sport, Estrada survived in freezing conditions after being swept from his yacht during a race. The 49-year-old sailor, who is lucky to be alive, was found by a tanker after his cries for help were heard. The tanker shielded Estrada while another yacht, the Victory, moved in, pulled him from the water, and treated him for shock. "They wrapped me in dry wool blankets and one of the guys jumped into the bunk with me and hung on to me, using his body temperature to warm me up," Estrada recounted.

By the time they reached land, Estrada had recovered sufficiently from his ordeal to help the crew moor the boat. However, at the press conference he seemed rather embarrassed by the attention.

The tanker captain who helped rescue Estrada said he hoped to catch up with the sailor in less dramatic circumstances. "He's an extremely lucky man," he said. "The next time I'm in San Diego I may call in to the Yacht Club to buy him a drink."

Estrada has been sailing since he was seven years old and ocean racing since the age of nineteen. But he confessed that after five hours alone in the sea, this was his last voyage.

b **GroupWork** Discussion. Compare your responses with 3 or 4 other students' responses. Were there any words or phrases that helped you to decide what was opinion?

c 🎧 Listen and note the similarities and differences between the newspaper report and the broadcast.

SIMILARITIES	DIFFERENCES

d What might be some reasons for the differences?

Task 3

a **GroupWork** Discussion. What is the most dramatic experience you have ever had? Describe it to the other students in the group.

b Decide on the most dramatic or interesting story.

c Have one group member tell that story to the class.

Language Focus 2 Relative adverbials: where/when/why/how

"I don't really understand how it happened."

Do you know the rule?

Fill in the chart using the words provided. The first one has been done for you.

how	in	manner
on	when	reason
for	why	during
time		

Preposition + which	Replaced by	Refers to
at, in, to, from	where	place
....	....	....
....	....	....
....	....	....

"Three a.m. was when they told Estrada's wife he was missing."

1 a Draw a line between the two parts of the sentences and join them with one of these words:

when	where	why	how

1 I don't really understand .... it came looking for me.
2 The place .... I saw the lights of a tanker coming towards me.
3 I saw the boat's lights .... they didn't see me was because of the huge waves.
4 The reason .... it happened was about 50 kilometers from shore.
5 It was around 5 a.m. ...*why*... it happened, but it did.

b Pair Work Practice the statements. *Student A:* Say the first part of the statement. *Student B:* Complete it.

2 Replace the underlined phrases with one of these words:

when	where	why	how

Example: <u>The way in which</u> the rescue happened was miraculous.
How the rescue happened was miraculous.

a The spot <u>at which</u> the accident happened was extremely remote.
....

b No one can understand <u>the way in which</u> the accident happened.
....

c Winter is the season <u>during which</u> most boating fatalities occur.
....

d The reports never explained <u>the reason for which</u> the tanker was moving towards the coast. ....

e <u>The manner in which</u> Estrada survived amazed everyone.
....

3 Group Work Think of something that happened to you recently. Tell the group when, where, how, and why the incident happened.

Language Focus 2: Relative adverbials:
where/ when/why/how

1. **(a)** Have students do this task individually. Circulate and give help if necessary. Elicit answers from around the class, and write them on the board. (Answers: 2. The place *where* it happened was about 50 kilometers from shore. 3. I saw the boat's lights *when* it came looking for me. 4. The reason *why* they didn't see me was because of the huge waves. 5. It was around 5 a.m. *when* I saw the lights of a tanker coming towards me.)

(b) Have students work in pairs, with the first student reading the beginning of each sentence and the second student adding the rest. Then have each student read the whole statement aloud.

2. Have students do this task individually and then work in pairs to compare and discuss their responses. Call on volunteers from around the class for answers. (Answers: b—how; c—when; d—why; e—How)

3. Students work in groups to recount a recent incident. Stress the need to include particulars—the when, where, etc. **Variation.** A second person in the group retells someone else's story immediately after that person has finished.

Do you know the rule?   This task involves students in actively thinking about how English works. Rather than providing the grammar rule for them, the exercise encourages students to use the examples to recognize language patterns and work out the rule for themselves.
(Answers: first column—during, for, in, manner, on; second column—how, when, why; third column—reason, time)

Self-Check

Communication Challenge

Challenge 2 is on pages 112, 114, and 116 of the student text, and instructions for its use are on page 112 in this Teacher's Extended Edition.

1, 2, 3.   Encourage students to complete the first three tasks without looking back at the unit.

4.   (a) Have students think of and write examples of language for giving short replies. Elicit responses from around the class.

(b) Students work in groups to brainstorm ideas for ways to practice using short replies. List these ideas on the board, and have students write them down.

5.   Have students make notes on who they will interview and what questions they will ask. Then have individuals report the stories they heard to the whole class.

6.   Have students work individually to check off the words that they know. **Optional.** Have each student exchange lists with a partner and then help each other with troublesome words.

•   Where do your students need additional help? Make a list for yourself. Decide how and where you can include this review/extension.

•   The grammar summary for this unit is on page 129. You may want to review this summary with your students.

Self-Check

COMMUNICATION CHALLENGE

Group Work Student A: Look at page 112. Student B: Look at page 114. Student C: Look at page 116.

1   Write down five new words you learned in this unit.

2   Write sentences using three of these new words.

3   Write three new sentences or questions you learned.

4 a

WHAT WOULD YOU SAY?

Someone tells you that they once saw a ghost.

You say:

Someone asks you about the most dramatic thing that ever happened to you.

You say:

b Group Work Brainstorm ways to practice this language out of class. Imagine you are visiting an English-speaking country. Where/When might you need this language?

5 Out of Class Interview friends, family, and acquaintances and find somebody who has had a strange experience. Report the story to the class. Who has the most interesting, unusual, or hard-to-believe story?

6   Vocabulary check. Check [√] the words you know.

Adjectives/Adverbs			Nouns			Verbs		
☐ believable	☐ mental	☐ spooky	☐ astral travel	☐ disbelief	☐ press	☐ account	☐ kid	☐ survive
☐ confused	☐ mysterious	☐ superstitious	☐ belief	☐ explanation	conference	☐ concentrate	☐ predict	
☐ crazy	☐ occasionally	☐ telepathic	☐ champion	☐ fiction	☐ shock	☐ interview	☐ shield	
☐ dramatic	☐ psychic	☐ unbelievable	☐ coincidence	☐ ghost	☐ similarity			
☐ freezing	☐ remote	☐ uncanny	☐ compulsion	☐ horoscope	☐ voyage			
☐ frightening	☐ rescued	☐ weird	☐ correlation	☐ junk food	☐ yacht			
☐ lucky	☐ spiritual							

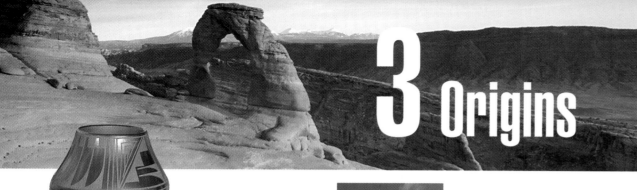

3 Origins

Warm-Up

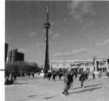
Canada

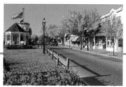
United States

Unit Goals

In this unit you will:

Emphasize information

"What makes my country special is the mix of nationalities."

"It's the mix of nationalities that makes my country special."

Talk about past events

"I went to Korea again last summer. I've been there twice now."

"I'd like to live in Thailand. It has a rich culture, great food, and wonderful people."

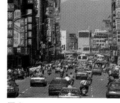
Japan Brazil

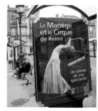
Taiwan France

1 a Group Work Brainstorm. Which of the countries pictured could these statements be about? (Note: There is no single correct answer for this task.)

1 What makes my country special is the fact that it is very safe, there is very little unemployment, and salaries are good.

2 What makes my country special is the sense of excitement. There's a lot of energy, and it affects everyone.

3 What makes my country special is the fact that our population is made up of people from many different parts of the world.

4 That's very simple. What makes my country special is the culture, the food, and the wine.

b Can you think of any other countries that match these statements?

2 a Would you like to live in another country for a while? Make a list of three countries you would like to live in and give reasons.

b Pair Work Share your list with another student.

Student text page 25

Warm-Up

This section provides a context for the unit. It presents the language of emphasizing information and talking about past events.

Unit Goals. Read each goal and sample language to the class. Ask students to circle the ones they can do in English. Ask a number of students for their responses to get an idea of the range in the group.

1. (a) Read through each statement with the whole class, or ask individual students to read them. Then have students work in groups to discuss which country they think is shown in each picture and which statement is the most appropriate for each picture. Circulate and make sure that students give reasons for their choices if there is disagreement.
(Answers: Accept reasonable responses. There is no single correct answer for the statements in this exercise.)
(b) Do this part as a brainstorm with the whole class.

2. (a) Working individually, students list three countries they would like to live in temporarily and give reasons for their choices.
(b) Students compare and discuss their choices with partners. Circulate and encourage students to use the sample language to *talk* about their choices rather than simply reading each other's papers.

Task Chain 1: People on the move

Task 1. With the whole class, read through each of the statements and make sure that everyone understands them. Then have students work in small groups to try to put the historical events in the order in which they happened. Students can order the events from most recent to earliest, or vice versa.
(Answers [1 = earliest; 5 = most recent]: 1—Spanish settlers; 2—British, French, etc.; 3—Revolutionary War; 4—European and Asian immigrants; 5—Spanish-speaking immigrants from Mexico and West Indies)

Task 2. Give students time to read the information and make notes on any information relating to the events mentioned in Task 1. Then have students check their answers. Elicit responses and questions from the whole class.

Learning Strategy. Personalizing means linking new learning to your life experiences and to your opinions, feelings, and ideas. Personalizing makes things relevant and meaningful, and it is essential for successful learning.

Task 3. (a) Brainstorm with the whole class four or five reasons why people emigrate to other countries. Then have students work in small groups to add any other reasons. **Optional.** You may want to extend the discussion by having students give reasons why certain people emigrate—for example, people who emigrate alone, with families, as young adults, in old age—and why emigrants choose the countries they do.

Task Chain 1 People on the move

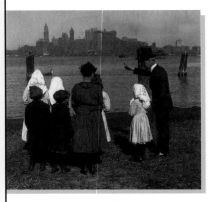

LEARNING STRATEGY
Personalizing = sharing your own opinions, feelings, and ideas about a subject.

"I think that most people emigrate for economic reasons."

Task 1

GroupWork How much do you know about U.S. history? Take this quiz to find out. Try to put these events in chronological order by numbering them 1 to 5.

.... Large numbers of Spanish-speaking people arrived from Mexico and the West Indies.
.... The English colonies rebelled against England in the Revolutionary War.
.... Spanish settlers arrived in Florida and Mexico.
.... Many British, French, Dutch, Germans, and Swedish people immigrated to the U.S.
.... Millions of immigrants arrived from Europe and Asia.

Task 2

Now check your answers to Task 1 by reading the following encyclopedia entry.

Immigration in the United States

First settled by "Indian" groups who migrated from Asia across the Bering land bridge over 25,000 years ago, the country was explored by the Norse (9th century), and by the Spanish (16th century) who settled in Florida and Mexico. In the 17th century there were settlements by the British, French, Dutch, Germans, and Swedish. Many Africans were introduced as slaves to work on the plantations. In the following century, British control grew throughout the area. A revolt of the English-speaking colonies in the War of Independence (1775-83) led to the creation of the United States of America.

In the 19th century millions of immigrants arrived from Europe and Asia, many of them refugees, leading to the description of the U.S.A. as a "melting pot" of nations. More recently, large numbers of Spanish-speaking people have arrived mainly from Central and South America.

Adapted from *Cambridge Encyclopedia*

Task 3

a **GroupWork** Brainstorm. Can you think of reasons why people emigrate?

b Think of one or two possible reasons for the following facts.

FACT	REASON(S)
In the 19th century, many people moved from Ireland to the U.S.	
Many people emigrated from Europe to Canada and the U.S. between 1946-56.	
Many people left the former Soviet Union in the 1920s.	
Many people left Hong Kong in the early 1990s.	
There was an increase in immigration to Australia in the 1950s and 60s.	
Many people left Lebanon during the 1980s.	

c Compare your reasons with another group.

Task 4

REASON	COUNTRY
1	
2	
3	
4	
5	

a 🎧 Listen to the lecture and list the reasons why people emigrate.

b 🎧 Listen again. What countries are mentioned in connection with each reason?

c Compare the responses you gave in Task 3 with the information in the lecture you just heard.

Task 5

You choose: Do Ⓐ or Ⓑ.

Ⓐ Make notes about the development of your own country. Answer questions such as:
- When did the population grow most quickly?
- Where did the people come from?
- Why did people emigrate from/immigrate to your country?

Group Work Tell your classmates about the development of your country.

Ⓑ The following is some information about the development of Canada. Based on the information, write a paragraph about the settlement of Canada.

IMMIGRATION TO CANADA

Thousands of Years Ago	Late 1700s	1763	Late 1800s	1945–early 1960s	1975–1985	1980s–early 1990s
Inuits, Indians	Scottish settlers	Quebec became part of Canada; 65,0000 French were living there	Other European immigrants arrived	After World War II, the greatest wave of immigration	113,000 refugees from Cambodia, Laos, Vietnam	Many immigrants from Hong Kong

---

(b) Discuss the first two facts with the whole class. Guide students to think about serious social changes such as war or famine as important reasons for emigration. Then have students work in small groups to complete the chart.
(Answers will vary.)

Have students write down their answers to 3a and 3b since they will need to refer to them again a little later in this section.

(c) Combine two or three groups, and have students compare and discuss their answers.

Task 4. **(a)** 🎧 Play the tape once. Have students listen for and note the reasons why people emigrate. Then play the tape a second time so that students can check their notes and then fill out the first column of the chart.
(Answers: poverty, hunger, hardship, opportunity, uncertainty)

(b) 🎧 Play the tape again. Students listen for and fill out the second column of the chart, matching each reason with the specific country.
(Answers: poverty—no country mentioned; hunger—Ireland; hardship—Soviet Union, Canada, United States; opportunity—Australia; uncertainty—Hong Kong, China)

(c) Students refer back to their responses in Tasks 3a and 3b, and compare these with the reasons given by the speakers.
(Answers will vary.)

Task 5. Students who choose **A** may need to consult an encyclopedia or find the information from some other source—for example, family members. Ask these students to do this in their own time, before the lesson. Then, in groups, they tell others about population trends in their own country.

Those who choose **B** can work in groups to produce the final paragraph. Have students read the passage individually and make notes. Then, working together, students summarize the information into one paragraph, writing a rough draft first. Correct spelling and grammar, and then have students write a second or final draft incorporating any corrections. Have students read their paragraph to other groups or to the whole class.

Language Focus 1: Present perfect & simple past

1. 🎧 Play the tape. Explain to students that the purpose of these conversations is to provide opportunities for speaking and pronunciation practice. In pairs, students practice the conversation. Have them practice line by line so they can say it from memory rather than reading it. **Variation.** Change the country, and have students fill in appropriate responses for Speaker B.

2. In pairs, students read the examples, then work together to fill in the missing verb tense for each of the sentences. Elicit answers from around the class.
(Answers: a—1. He *enjoyed* it so much that he plans to return next year. 2. He *has shown* us his slide collection five times since his return. b—1. She *fell* in love with her third husband at first sight. 2. She *has not been* so happy since her second husband left. c—1. Kanya is my best friend, although I *have not* seen her for weeks. 2. . . . *did not* like her very much when I first met her. d—1. They *have regretted* the decision ever since they moved. 2. They originally *went* there for a vacation.)

3. Have students do this task individually. Circulate and offer assistance if necessary.
(Answers: a—have been; b—missed; c—have decided; d—did not see; e—haven't been)

Do you know the rule? Students work individually to match the rule with the examples.
(Answers: 1—c, PP; 2—b, SP; 3—a, PP)

Language Focus 1 Present perfect & simple past

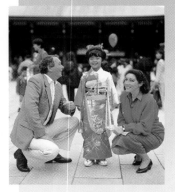

1 🎧 **Pair Work** Listen. Then practice the conversation.

A: Why did you decide to go to Japan?
B: I've always been fascinated by Japanese culture and I've read a lot about the country and its people, and I wanted to see it for myself.
A: And what did you think?
B: Well, it was the most incredible experience I've ever had.

2 **Pair Work** Complete these statements using the present perfect (*have lived*) for one statement and the simple past tense (*lived*) for the other statement.

Example: Lilly and Jo are fluent in Portuguese, even though they . . .
1 *have never lived* (never live) in a Portuguese-speaking country.
2 *didn't learn* (not learn) it until they were in their twenties.

a Tom made his first visit to Japan last year.
1 He .... (enjoy) it so much that he plans to return next year.
2 He .... (show) us his slide collection five times since his return.

b It was Sylvia's mother's third marriage.
1 She .... (fall) in love with her third husband at first sight.
2 She .... (not be) so happy since her second husband left.

c Kanya is my best friend, although I . . .
1 .... (not see) her for weeks.
2 .... (not like) her very much when I first met her.

d They finally settled in Australia two years ago.
1 They .... (regret) the decision ever since they moved.
2 They originally .... (go) there for a vacation.

3 Fill in the blanks with an appropriate form of the verb in parentheses.
a We .... (be) at the party since it started.
b We .... (miss) the concert because we didn't get tickets.
c Since that wild party last week, I .... (decide) I'm not the party type.
d I .... (not see) you at Paul's place last week.
e I .... (not go) to a party since my brother's birthday.

Do you know the rule?

Match the uses of the simple past and present perfect with the examples by writing a letter under "example." Indicate which tense, simple past (SP) or present perfect (PP) is being referred to by writing SP or PP under "Tense."

Uses	Example	Tense
1 A state continuing from past to present.	....	....
2 Completed events at a definite time in the past.	....	....
3 Habits or recurring events in a period leading to the present.	....	....

Examples:
a I've been to ten parties in the last month.
b She didn't come to the party because she was sick.
c We've been here for hours.

Task Chain 2 A sense of identity

"Living in another country is really exciting because it gives you an opportunity to learn about another culture."

Task 1

a Group Work Brainstorm. Make a list of the good things and the bad things about living in another country.

Good Things	Bad Things
....	....
....	....
....	....

b Group Work Now take turns making statements following the model.

Task 2

a 🎧 Listen. You will hear Dave, Anne, and Denise talking about what it's like to live in another country. None of them live in the country where they were born. Make a note of the places you hear.

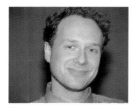
Dave

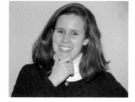
Denise

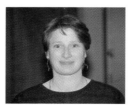
Anne

b 🎧 Group Work Listen again. Where were these three people born? Where are they living now? Use the information on the tape and the fact sheet at left to fill in the chart.

NAME	WHERE FROM	WHERE LIVING NOW
Anne		
Denise		
Dave		

c Group Work Discussion. What does each person say about "culture"?

NAME	TOPIC	COMMENT
Anne	British culture	
Denise	California culture	
Dave	Popular culture	

d 🎧 Listen to the tape again to check your answers.

Task Chain 2: A sense of identity

Task 1. (a) In small groups, students list good and bad things about living in another country. Encourage them to think of their own experiences and those of anyone they know who has lived for a time in another country. **Variation.** Ask three or four others in the class for their ideas about living in another country. Then have the groups compare and discuss the responses each student has offered.

(b) Using the examples discussed in Task 1a, have each student in the group practice making at least one statement. Remind them to use the sample language. Circulate and monitor pronunciation and content. **Variation.** Give students time to memorize one of the statements made in their group. Then call on at least one student from each group to make their statement to the whole class, without reading.

Task 2. (a) 🎧 Play the tape. Students listen individually and write down the places mentioned by Dave, Anne, and Denise. Elicit answers at random from around the class.
(Answers: Dave—Australia, Canada; Anne—Britain, Australia; Denise—California, Australia)

(b) 🎧 In small groups, students first read the fact sheet and then examine the table they are to fill in. Play the tape again. Students listen, make notes, and then fill out the table.
(Answers: Anne—Britain, Australia; Denise—Australia, California; Dave—Canada, Australia)

(c) This is a selective listening task. Have students, in groups, discuss what each speaker says about culture. Elicit answers from around the class.
(Answers: Anne—comes from a culture where her background is known; Denise—people don't care about her background; Dave—is ignorant about popular culture)

(d) 🎧 Successful listening involves predicting and then verifying predictions. This task allows students to check their personal predictions by listening to the tape and to discuss how their predictions were different from those of other students. Have students also discuss which of their predictions were right.

Task 3. Discuss with the class the strategy of inferring. Have the students first read the extracts individually and mark any words or phrases that help them infer who wrote the letter.
(Answers: first extract—Dave; second extract—Denise; third extract—Anne)

Task 4. (a) Students prepare for this task by choosing a country they have visited or know about. With the whole class, discuss the format of the letter, and have students brainstorm what they will describe in their letters—for example, the cities, the people, natural scenery, customs. Have students limit the letter to a single paragraph. **Variation.** Prepare a model of a letter and write it on an overhead or on the board for students to refer to as they are writing.
(b) Have students exchange letters and try to guess which country is being described.

Task 5. If the students are all from the same country, have them do **A** or **B** in small groups. Encourage students who choose **A** to think of real-life examples of visitors' comments, either things they have heard or comments they have read. Tell students who choose **B** to think first about how they would describe their country or culture—that is, what things are common or even unique in their culture. Then they make a list of these.

Task 3

The following excerpts are from letters written by Anne, Denise, and Dave to friends and family back home not long after they began living in their new country. Who wrote which letter?

Excerpts   *Written by*

I had dinner with my new boss last night. It was interesting, although rather confusing. The conversation was all about movies I'd never seen, writers I'd never read, and singers I'd never heard of.   ....

Physically the country is about the same size, but in every other respect, the differences are simply overwhelming. There are twice as many people in this state than in our whole country.   ....

I've had an interesting time since I arrived. I was invited to my first party on Saturday night, and it was great fun, although I spent the entire evening telling my story over and over, which got a bit frustrating.   ....

Task 4

a Pick a country and write an imaginary letter to friends at home. Don't mention the country.

b **Pair Work** Exchange letters and try and guess the country your partner wrote about.

Dear All,
I'm still having a fabulous time. I've just come back from a week camping in the desert. It was ....

....

Task 5

You choose: Do **A** or **B**.

A **Pair Work** Make a list of the things that visitors would say about *your* country.

B Make a list of the things that give your country a sense of identity (famous people, significant events in history, etc.).

"Believe it or not, the thing that gives my country a sense of identity is the fact that it's made up of people from all over the world."

Language Focus 2 Emphasis with *it* & *what*

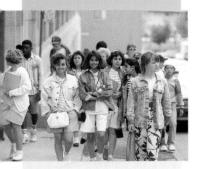

1 🎧 **Pair Work** Listen. Then practice the conversation using information that is true for you.

A: What makes Canada special for you, Dave?

B: I guess it's the tolerance of the people that makes the place special for me. What also makes it special is the mix of nationalities. We have people here from all over the world. What about you?

A: Well, what makes Australia special is that it's at the end of the earth, so it's still relatively innocent. I guess it's also the mix of people from all over the world. I guess we're a bit like Canada from that perspective.

2 Rewrite these statements. Begin with *what* or *it's*.

Example: It's the lack of unemployment that makes my country special.

What *makes my country special is the lack of unemployment.*

a What makes my country special is the fact that it is very safe.

It's ....

b It's the sense of excitement that makes my country interesting.

What ....

c What makes my country special is the political freedom.

It's ....

d It's the culture, the food, and the wine that make my country unique.

What ....

e What makes my country important is the fact that I was born there!

It's ....

A What I hate about my school is the amount of traveling to get there.

B It's the traveling to get there that Yumi hates about her school.

3 a **Pair Work** Say what you . . .

like . . .	about your	. . . country
dislike		school
love		friends
admire		etc.

b Report what your partner says to another pair.

Language Focus 2: Emphasis with *it* & *what*

1. 🎧 Play the tape. Then have students think about and write down two or three things they find special about their own country. Read through the conversation with the whole class, and note those parts that will need to be changed to make the information true for them. Have pairs of students practice the conversation line by line, memorizing the lines so that in the end they can deliver the whole conversation from memory rather than having to read it. Circulate and monitor content, grammar, and pronunciation.

2. Have students do this task individually. (Answers: a—It's the fact that my country is very safe that makes it special. b—What makes my country interesting is the sense of excitement. c—It's the political freedom that makes my country special. d—What makes my country unique is the culture, the food, and the wine. e—It's the fact that I was born there that makes my country special!)

3. **(a)** With the whole class, brainstorm four or five new categories of things to like or dislike. Then have students work in pairs to discuss what they like and dislike about their own country. Remind students of the importance of discussions such as these, in which they link the learning to their own experience and opinions.

   (b) Combine pairs and have students report what their partner said. Circulate and monitor grammar and pronunciation.

Self-Check

Communication Challenge

Challenge 3 is on page 112 of the student text, and suggestions for its use are on that page in this Teacher's Extended Edition.

In the Self-Check tasks, students rate their own progress on the tasks in the unit. As much as possible, these tasks should be done out of class and then discussed in a general feedback session.

1, 2, 3. Encourage students to complete the first three tasks without looking back at the unit.

4. (a) Have students work individually to think of and write examples of language for asking about and describing places. They then produce a statement describing their country, a question about the special qualities of a friend's hometown, and a statement listing some of the places they've visited. Elicit responses from around the class.

(b) In groups, students brainstorm ideas for practicing the language of describing places and asking others to describe places. Call on each group to give at least two ideas. List these on the board, and have students write them down.

5. Tasks such as this one are designed to develop independent learning skills. Students have to gather information and find out more about specific issues. This involves speaking practice and gives opportunities for students to be involved in meaningful communication with others. Encourage students to compile a list of the exact questions they will ask the people they interview *before* the actual interviews.

6. Have students work individually to check off the words that they know.

• The grammar summary for this unit is on page 130.

Self-Check

COMMUNICATION CHALLENGE

Pair Work Look at Challenge 3 on page 112.

1 Write down five new words you learned in this unit.

....

2 Write sentences using three of these new words.

....

....

....

3 Write three new sentences or questions you learned.

....

....

....

4 a

WHAT WOULD YOU SAY?

Someone asks you what makes your country special.

You say: ....

You want to know what makes a friend's hometown special.

You say: ....

Someone asks you what places you've visited.

You say: ....

b **Group Work** Brainstorm ways to practice this language out of class. Imagine you are visiting an English-speaking country. Where/When might you need this language?

5 **Out of Class** Talk to three people who have immigrated to your country from another country or who have spent time living in another country. Ask them about their experiences and report back to the class.

6 Vocabulary check. Check [√] the words you know.

Adjectives/Adverbs			Nouns			Verbs		
☐ confusing	☐ overwhelming	☐ safe	☐ consulate	☐ immigrant	☐ salary	☐ emigrate	☐ immigrate	☐ regret
☐ crazy	☐ political	☐ simple	☐ creation	☐ immigration	☐ settlement	☐ emphasize	☐ introduce	
☐ frustrating	☐ practical	☐ unique	☐ culture	☐ mix	☐ slave	☐ explore	☐ personalize	
☐ incredible	☐ relatively		☐ encyclopedia	☐ perspective	☐ tolerance			
☐ innocent	☐ rich		☐ history	☐ population	☐ unemployment			
			☐ identity	☐ revolt				

4 Good Advice

Warm-Up

Unit Goals

In this unit you will:

Ask for and give advice

"If you stay up late at night, you should take a nap during the day."

"What should I do when I can't get to sleep at night?"

Express preferences

"I prefer people who are neat."

"I dislike people whose friends stay up talking half the night."

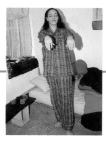
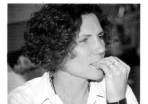
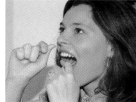
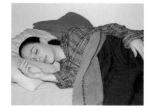

1 a Look at the pictures and make a list of the habits you see.

b Group Work Brainstorm. Make a list of group members' good and bad habits.

NAME	GOOD HABITS	BAD HABITS

c Group Work Compare them with another group. Do your good habits seem better than those of the other group? Do their bad habits seem worse than yours?

d Group Work Discussion. What are habits? Why do we have habits?

2 Group Work Listen and discuss. What habit is the speaker talking about? Do you think the habit is normal or rather unusual? Why?

Good Advice **33**

Warm-Up

Unit Goals. This section presents the language of asking for and giving advice, and expressing preferences. Read out each goal and sample language, or have individual students read them. Have students circle those they can do in English.

1. (**a**) Discuss with the class the concept of habits as behavior patterns.

(**b**) Start the discussion by presenting the idea that good habits often result from knowledge or training, and bad habits are more often unconscious behaviors. Give students time to think about their own habits and to list them under two headings—Good Habits and Bad Habits. Stress that in different communities there will be different opinions about what kinds of habits are good or bad. In small groups, students then discuss their lists and from these compile a list of their group's habits.

(**c**) Combine two or three groups to discuss and compare answers.

(**d**) Introduce the discussion by mentioning that habits are behavior patterns that we do not think about. We fall into our habits automatically. Make this a controlled discussion with the whole class. Manage the discussion so that the most talkative students do not dominate. Call on those students who usually talk less to give their personal views and opinions. The objective of the discussion is to share ideas and opinions, not to arrive at consensus.

2. Play the tape. In groups, students listen for the habit the speaker is talking about, and then they discuss how this habit would be viewed in their country or culture.
(Answer: napping)

Good Advice **33**

Task Chain 1: A good night's rest

Task 1. Read through the true/false statements with the whole class. Then have students work in groups to respond to each one. It is important to give learners opportunities to voice their opinions, based on their own knowledge and experience, and to hear those of others.
(Answers to the quiz will vary.)

Task 2. (a) Before students brainstorm suggestions, each group should first determine exactly what the sleeping problem is. Then they brainstorm various pointers to help the person sleep better. **Optional.** Have each student practice giving advice by using at least one suggestion from his or her list of advice and using the sample language as a model.

(b) 🎧 With the whole class, read through the list of possible causes and explain any, if necessary. Play the tape. Working individually, students listen and fill in the first three columns of the chart.
(Answers: worry about work—yes; soft mattress—not sure; irregular bedtime—yes; lack of exercise—yes; eating a large meal—no; being a smoker—not sure; drinking coffee—yes)

(c) 🎧 Play the tape again. Have students listen this time for the advice given in each case.
(Answers: worry about work—set planning time earlier in the evening; irregular bedtime—establish regular pattern; lack of exercise—engage in regular exercise; drinking coffee—avoid)

(d) 🎧 Have students work in groups—if possible, the same groups as they were in for Task 1. Give them time to reread the true/false list. Then play the tape and have students check which of the statements from the list are mentioned.
(Answers: c, f)

Task 1

Group Work Quiz. How do you feel about sleep? Decide whether the statements below are true or false.

Sleep Quiz	True	False
a. Sleeping during the day is bad for you.	....	....
b. Adults do not need more than six hours' sleep.	....	....
c. Jogging during the day will help you sleep better at night.	....	....
d. Eating a large evening meal can help you sleep.	....	....
e. People who smoke are heavier sleepers than non-smokers.	....	....
f. Going to bed at the same time every night helps us sleep better.	....	....
g. Firm mattresses provide better rest than soft ones.	....	....
h. Going to bed without eating can cause sleeplessness.	....	....

Task 2

a **Group Work** Brainstorm suggestions for helping someone who has trouble sleeping.

b 🎧 You will hear someone getting advice about her sleep problems. Listen and check [√] the things that are causing her difficulty.

	YES	NO	NOT SURE	ADVICE
Worry about work				
Soft mattress	.			
Going to bed at irregular hours				
Lack of exercise				
Eating a large meal				
Being a smoker				
Drinking coffee				

c 🎧 Listen again. In the last column make a note of any advice that is given.

d 🎧 **Group Work** Which of the true/false items in Task 1 are mentioned in the conversation? Listen once more and check your group's answers to Task 1.

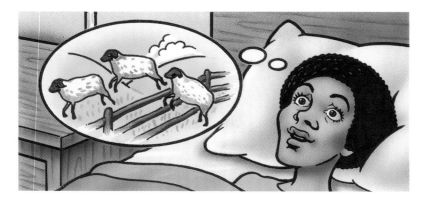

"I heard that counting sheep was supposed to help."

"Both the conversation and the article mention keeping regular hours. The article talks about sleeping on a good bed."

Task 3

a Read the following article and underline the information that was discussed in the conversation in Task 2. Make a list of the new information.

b **Pair Work** Compare your responses with another student.

You *Can* Get a Good Night's Rest!

Nothing is more essential to a good day than a good night's sleep. But on any given night, one in three people has difficulty sleeping and most of us get less sleep than we need. Increasing your comfort while sleeping can be important in helping you get a good night's rest. According to Andrea Herman, director of the Better Sleep Council, "We sometimes sacrifice sleep because of our busy lifestyles. That makes the sleep we do get even more important." Herman suggests you do the following to improve the quality of your sleep.

- **Keep regular hours.** Try to get up at the same time every morning regardless of how much or how little sleep you've had.
- **Exercise regularly.** Taking a 30-minute walk, jogging, or swimming three or four times a week will help you sleep better and deeper.
- **Cut down on caffeine.** This drug, found in coffee, cola, and tea can interfere with sleep. "Drink your last cup of coffee no later than six to eight hours before your usual bedtime," says Herman.
- **Sleep on a good bed.** "It's difficult to get a good night's rest on a bed that's too small, too hard, or too soft."
- **Don't smoke.** Studies have found that heavy smokers awaken more times during the night and spend less time in deep sleep than non-smokers.
- **Go for quality, not quantity.** Six hours of deep, solid sleep will make you feel more rested than eight hours of light, interrupted sleep.
- **Set aside a "worry" or planning time early in the evening.** To keep from rehearsing your plans or problems while your head's on the pillow, make a list of things to do and of your concerns before you go to bed.
- **Don't go to bed stuffed or starved.** Heavy, high-fat meals may make you feel drowsy at first, but they can keep you tossing and turning all night. Likewise, your grumbling stomach may prevent deep sleep if you go to bed hungry.
- **Develop a sleep ritual.** Children often benefit from repeating a calming sleep ritual. Adults also can benefit from a ritual—doing easy stretches, reading a book, taking a warm bath, or listening to music.

Source: Adapted from *Vitality*, August 1994

Task 4

a Survey. Complete the following survey on sleep habits.

	Always	Often	Hardly ever	Never
1 I go to bed at the same time every night.	....	....	....	....
2 I am asleep by 10:30 P.M.	....	....	....	....
3 I am still up at 1 A.M.	....	....	....	....
4 I find it difficult to get to sleep.	....	....	....	....
5 I lie awake worrying about things.	....	....	....	....
6 I take a nap during the day.	....	....	....	....
7 I sleep for more than eight hours.	....	....	....	....

b **Group Work** Now interview two other students.

c **Group Work** Discussion. Which members of the class get the most sleep? The least? Why?

Task 3. (a) If necessary, replay the tape from Task 2. Have students do this task individually. Students scan the article and note any information that they heard in the conversation. Play the tape again and have students underline information in the article that is mentioned on the tape and make a list of any information in the article that was not heard in the conversation. (Answers: Same—exercise regularly; cut down on caffeine; set aside a "worry" or planning time early in the evening; don't go to bed stuffed or starved. New—keep regular hours; sleep on a good bed; don't smoke; go for quality, not quantity; develop a sleep ritual.)

(b) Have each student compare and discuss responses with another student. Circulate and check pronunciation. Make sure that students use the sample language as a model.

Task 4. (a) Remind students that the main purposes of a survey are to gather information and practice speaking. In the classroom, surveys help learners find out more about one another, and they also create a friendly and supportive learning environment. Have each student answer the survey questions.

(b) In small groups, students compare and discuss their responses.

(c) In a whole-class discussion, have students figure out from the survey answers those members of the class who get the most sleep and those who get the least.

Language Focus 1: *When* and *if* clauses + modal *should/shouldn't*

1. 🎧 Play the tape. Have students listen and follow the text. Then model the conversation with one or two students from the class. With the whole class, practice the conversation. Then have students practice in pairs so they learn the conversation and can say it from memory.

2. Do the first sentence with the whole class. Write the beginning of the sentence on the board and have students suggest possible endings: "If you find yourself sitting next to someone in a restaurant whose smoking bothers you, you should . . . (ask the person to stop, ask to speak to the manager, etc.)." Then have students work to complete the other sentences. Circulate and correct spelling and grammar. Elicit answers from around the class.

Learning Strategy. Discuss with students the fact that finding patterns in language helps the reading process. Link this concept to predicting.

3. Do the first sentence with the whole class: "When you have trouble getting to sleep at night, you should . . . (try to complete a task left over from the day, do light exercises, etc.)." Then have students work in pairs to discuss what advice they would give in each case and complete the sentence. Circulate and correct spelling and grammar.

4. (a) With the whole class, list the things people have received advice on so far in this unit—for example, trouble sleeping, noisy roommate, partner who snores, trouble getting up. Then ask students for issues on which they would like advice, and discuss this list with the class.
    (b) With the whole class, decide which request for advice was most interesting/unusual/creative.

Do you know the rule? Students are encouraged to use examples and models to recognize language patterns and work out grammar/language rules for themselves. (Answers: *when—are going to; if—might*)

Language Focus 1 *When* and *if* clauses + modal *should/shouldn't*

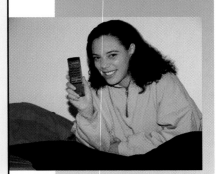

1 🎧 **Pair Work** Listen to the conversation. Then practice it with a partner.

A: My sister and her husband are coming to visit this weekend.
B: Oh, that's great!
A: Well, it's good and bad. She's very messy, and he's an insomniac.
B: A *what*?
A: An insomniac—someone who has trouble sleeping. He spends most of the night watching TV and keeping everyone else awake.
B: Oh, no.
A: What should I do if she leaves her stuff all over the place?
B: If she leaves her clothes all over the place, you should put them in a bag and send them to the most expensive cleaner in town.
A: What a great idea! And what should I do when her husband keeps us all awake?
B: When you go to bed, take the TV remote control with you.
A: What a great idea!

Do you know the rule?

Complete the following statements by circling the correct alternative.

We use *when* in talking about events that *are going to / might* happen.

We use *if* in talking about events that *are going to / might* happen.

LEARNING STRATEGY

Discovering = finding patterns in language.

"Before you go to bed, you should take a bubble bath."

2 **Pair Work** Complete these sentences using *if* or *when*. Then practice making statements and responding to them.

Example:
You win a lot of money. → If you win a lot of money, you should always give some to charity. It brings good luck.

a In a restaurant, you find yourself sitting next to someone whose smoking bothers you.
b You get a low grade on an exam.
c You meet someone for the first time.
d Someone you know well gets married.
e Someone you know well has an accident.

3 **Pair Work** What advice would you give to someone . . .

a who has trouble getting to sleep at night?
b whose roommate stays up until very late listening to loud music?
c whose partner snores in their sleep?
d who has trouble getting up in the morning?

4 a **Group Work** Make a list of five or six things you would like advice on. Now circulate and take turns with other students asking for advice.

b **Group Work** Discussion. Who had the most interesting/unusual request for advice? Who had the most creative/unusual advice to give?

Task Chain 2 Kicking the habit

"I'm always interrupting others in conversation. This is a really annoying habit that I'd like to change."

Task 1

a **Group Work** Discussion. Have you ever tried to quit a bad habit? Do you know anyone else who has? What methods did you/they use? Were the methods successful? Why or why not?

b **Pair Work** Study the following statements and decide how each person gave up their bad habit. Write the number of the method in the blank.

1 support groups   3 physician's advice   5 cold turkey
2 hypnosis   4 self-help approaches

.... "I tried quitting by myself, but it didn't work. I finally went to see our family doctor."

.... "I bought a book and a tape, and managed to cure myself."

.... "Every Tuesday and Thursday, I went over to our local community center and met with five or six other people who were also trying to quit. We'd talk and give each other help and advice."

.... "It worked the very first time. I had to lie down and close my eyes, relax, and just listen to the therapist. I never had the urge to raid the cookie jar again."

.... "I just got up one morning and said to myself, 'That's it!' I stopped completely, just like that. It's the only way to do it."

c Skim the magazine article. Which of these types of support are referred to in the article? Write yes or no in the first column of the chart on page 38.

Kick the Habit

There are numerous ways of giving up bad habits, although not all are equally effective for all habits and all people. The secret of successfully ridding oneself of a bad habit is to match the method, the habit, and one's own personality. Going cold turkey might be fine for someone with an iron will and intense motivation, but not for the person who thinks that success should come in small, achievable steps. Hypnosis might work for someone who wants to quit smoking, or who has an eating disorder, but is probably inappropriate for someone who wants to stop biting their nails. Type of habit and personality will also determine the amount of support that someone will need. Some people are readily able to take advantage of the various self-help options available, while others will need the assistance of support groups in order to kick their habit successfully.

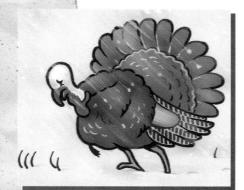

Task Chain 2: Kicking the habit

Task 1. **(a)** Students think about their own habits and choose one they would like to change. Then, in small groups, students compare and discuss the bad habits they have chosen. Have students tell the class their bad habits, and then list these on the board. (You will need to record these since they are referred to again in Task 3.) The class brainstorms possible ways of changing the habits. Make this a controlled discussion with the whole class. Manage the discussion so that each of the questions is discussed. Call on those students who usually talk less to give their opinions. **Variation.** Have students prepare for this task before the lesson.

(b) With the whole class, go through the list of support types and explain any that students do not know. Remind students that there are different ways of reading, depending on the reason for reading. In this case, it is very important for language learners to read carefully for detail. Have students work in pairs to read the article. They then fill in the type of support. Circulate and provide assistance if necessary. (Answers: 3, 4, 1, 2, 5)

(c) Have students read the article and then fill in the first column of the chart on page 37. (Answers, top to bottom: yes, yes, no, yes, yes)

(d) Have students work in groups to brainstorm a habit that might be effectively dealt with by each method and then fill in the second column of the chart. (Answers will vary.)

(e) Students work in the same groups to come up with particular advantages and disadvantages of the five methods and then fill in the last two columns of the chart. At this point, have them exchange charts with another group to compare and discuss. (Answers will vary but should reflect the information in the article.)

Task 2. **(a)** 🎧 Play the tape. Working individually, students listen and then write in the chart the callers' habits and unsuccessful ways of dealing with them. (Answers: Camilla—daughter's nail-biting; put bad-tasting material on daughter's hands. Tom—junk food; tried appetite suppressants. Melissa—brother's weird noises; complained to parents.)

(b) 🎧 Play the tape again. This time, students listen for the suggestions offered to the callers and complete the chart. (Answers: Camilla—monetary reward; Tom—Overeaters Anonymous; Melissa—tape-record brother's noises)

(c) 🎧 Play the tape once more. Have students listen and then work in pairs to compare and confirm their responses.

(d) Students work in small groups to analyze the suggestions and to try to improve on them.

Task 3. If students choose **A**, have them work in pairs, using the sample language to ask for and offer advice. Students who choose **B** should first work individually to create the list of annoying habits. Then, in pairs, they share their lists and try to find ways to help their friends/family eliminate the bad habits. Have them use the sample language to present each solution. Then each pair discusses solutions with another pair.

METHOD	REFERRED TO? (YES OR NO)	HABITS	ADVANTAGES	DISADVANTAGES
support groups				
hypnosis				
physician advice				
self-help approaches				
cold turkey				

d Group Work Brainstorm. What habits do you think each method is suited to? Fill in the second column in the chart.

e Group Work What are some advantages and disadvantages of the different methods? Complete the chart, then compare with another group.

Task 2

a 🎧 Listen to the radio call-in show. People are asking for advice on how to kick a habit or how to help someone else to kick a bad habit. In the chart, fill in the habit and the people's unsuccessful methods of quitting.

b 🎧 Listen again and write the suggestions in the chart.

PERSON	HABIT	UNSUCCESSFUL METHOD	SUGGESTION
Camilla			
Tom			
Melissa			

c 🎧 Pair Work Check your responses with another student.

d Group Work Do you think that these suggestions are good ones? Can you think of better suggestions?

Task 3

You choose: Do **A** or **B**.

A Look at the bad habit you listed in Task 1. Ask your partner for advice on how to kick the habit.

B Make a list of habits family members or friends have that annoy you.

Pair Work Think of ways to encourage the people to quit their bad habits. Write them down.

Group Work Discuss your solutions with another pair.

A I want to quit smoking. What should I do?

B Why don't you go cold turkey? That worked for me.

"My friend David is a workaholic. I think he needs to take a vacation every year."

Language Focus 2 Relative clauses with *whose/who/who is*

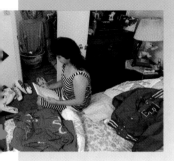

1 🎧 Listen to the conversation between Mitch and Lisa and complete these statements.

a Lisa likes people who ....

b Lisa doesn't like people whose ....

c Lisa would like to live with someone who's ....

d Mitch likes people whose ....

e Mitch doesn't like people who ....

Who would you like to share a house/apartment with?

	You			Your Partner		
	Y	N	D	Y	N	D
someone who smokes	☐	☐	☐	☐	☐	☐
someone who's a messy cook	☐	☐	☐	☐	☐	☐
someone whose parties go on all night	☐	☐	☐	☐	☐	☐
someone who plays classical music	☐	☐	☐	☐	☐	☐
someone whose relatives are always visiting	☐	☐	☐	☐	☐	☐
someone who's extremely neat	☐	☐	☐	☐	☐	☐
someone who stays home a lot	☐	☐	☐	☐	☐	☐
someone who gets up very early	☐	☐	☐	☐	☐	☐
someone whose boss calls all the time	☐	☐	☐	☐	☐	☐
....	☐	☐	☐	☐	☐	☐
....	☐	☐	☐	☐	☐	☐

2 a Complete the survey at left by checking the appropriate box [√] in column 1.

Key: Y = yes
N = no
D = don't care

b **Pair Work** Now add two items to the list, and then survey a partner on the entire list.

c **Pair Work** Now tell someone else about your partner's preferences.

A "Shelly, would you like to live with someone who goes out a lot?"

B "I don't care."

A (to C) "Shelly doesn't care if she lives with someone who goes out a lot."

Do you know the rule?

Group Work Discussion. When do we use who's and whose?

3 Combine these sentences using *who*, *who's*, or *whose* and practice them.

a We met some friends at a café. They invited us to a late night party.

b We met some students at the party. Their roommate is moving out.

c I like certain people. Particularly those who are considerate of others.

d I am bored by certain people. Particularly those with limited interests.

e I can't stand certain people. Particularly when they interrupt all the time.

Language Focus 2: Relative clauses with *whose/who/who is*

1. 🎧 Explain to students that when we listen and understand something, we recall the meaning of what was said, but not usually the exact words that we heard. Play the tape. Have students do this task individually. Elicit answers at random from around the class.
(Answers: a—people who are neat; b—idea of a good time is to stay up late and make a lot of noise; c—away most of the time; d—attitude is considerate; e—only think of themselves)

2. (a) Read through the survey questions with the whole class. Then have each student answer the questions.
(b) Each student adds two items to the list and then surveys his or her partner. Circulate and give assistance as necessary.
(c) Have students find a new partner and tell him or her the responses of the first partner. Circulate and monitor pronunciation.

3. It is important to give learners opportunities to make intelligent guesses about English and how it works. Have students, in groups, share how they think the sentences should be combined and why they think so. Then have students complete the exercise individually. Direct them to the sample language.
(Answers: a—We met some friends at a café who invited . . .; b—We met some students at the party whose roommate . . .; c—I like certain people, particularly those who are . . .; d—I am bored with certain people, particularly those who have limited . . .; e—I can't stand certain people, particularly those who interrupt . . .)

Do you know the rule? Have students work in small groups to try to infer the rule for using *who's* and *whose*. Refer them to their answers in the combining exercise.

Self-Check

Communication Challenge

Challenge 4 is on page 113 of the student text, and suggestions for its use are on that page in this Teacher's Extended Edition.

1, 2, 3. Encourage students to complete the first three tasks without looking back at the unit.

4. (a) Individually, students think of and write examples of language for asking for and giving advice and expressing preferences. **Optional.** Have them compare their responses with another student. Elicit responses from the class.
(b) In small groups, students brainstorm ideas about when/where they might need to ask for and give advice, and express preferences. Circulate and make sure the suggestions are as specific as possible. Encourage students to think about situations they have been in when they needed to use this kind of language.

5. Encourage students to compile a list of the exact questions they will ask *before* they carry out the interview. If possible, have students do this task in English; if not, they can perform the interviews in their first language and then report to the class in English.

6. Have students work individually to check off the words that they know.

• The grammar summary for this unit is on page 130.

Self-Check

COMMUNICATION CHALLENGE

Look at Challenge 4 on page 113.

"Well, I'd probably need to ask for advice."

1 Write down five new words you learned in this unit.

....

2 Write sentences using three of these new words.

....

....

3 Write three new sentences or questions you learned.

....

....

4 a

WHAT WOULD YOU SAY?

You want some advice on sleeping better.
You say: ....

Someone asks for your advice on quitting smoking.
You say: ....

Someone asks you whether you prefer people who stay up late or people who go to bed early.
You say: ....

b **Group Work** Brainstorm ways to practice this language out of class. Imagine you are visiting an English-speaking country. Where/When might you need this language?

5 **Out of Class** Interview three people about someone they have lived with. Find out three good things and three not-so-good things and make notes. Bring the information to your next class and discuss it.

6 Vocabulary check. Check [√] the words you know.

Adjectives/Adverbs			Nouns			Verbs		Modals
☐ calming	☐ inappropriate	☐ often	☐ acupuncture	☐ hypnosis	☐ quantity	☐ compare	☐ quit	☐ might
☐ creative	☐ individual	☐ regularly	☐ advice	☐ insomniac	☐ ritual	☐ cure	☐ rest	☐ should
☐ essential	☐ irregular	☐ self-help	☐ caffeine	☐ motivation	☐ sleeplessness	☐ determine	☐ sacrifice	☐ shouldn't
☐ grumbling	☐ never	☐ trouble	☐ charity	☐ nap	☐ therapist	☐ dislike	☐ worry	
☐ hardly ever	☐ normal	☐ unusual	☐ comfort	☐ options	☐ workaholic	☐ encourage		
			☐ community center	☐ preferences		☐ kick		
				☐ quality		☐ prefer		

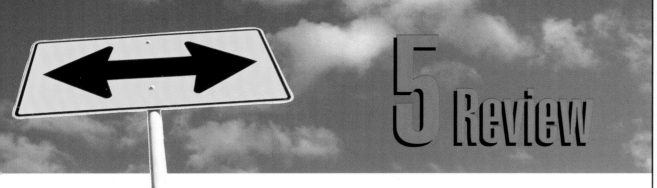

5 Review

Task 1

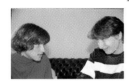

Picture 1

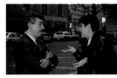

Picture 2

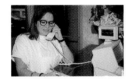

Picture 3

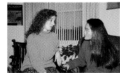

Picture 4

a Use your imagination. Look at the pictures and decide which person is doing the following things. Write the number of the picture in the blank.

.... requesting information   .... giving advice
.... expressing disbelief   .... making an excuse

b **Pair Work** Compare responses with another student, giving reasons for your choices.

Task 2

a Look at these functions. Match them with the pieces of conversation listed below. Write the correct number in the blank.

.... requesting information
...../... expressing disbelief
.... issuing an invitation
.... giving advice
.... responding to an invitation
.... expressing a preference

1 You're kidding me!
2 Well, next time he does it, I would . . .
3 I'm just calling up to see if you can . . .
4 Could you tell me where the . . .
5 You might like . . . but I like people who . . .
6 I would love to!

b **Pair Work** Think of a situation for each of these pieces of conversation. Make up two-line dialogues and practice them with a partner.

Task 3

A My brother insists on smoking in the apartment, even though he knows I hate it.

B Well, next time he does it, I would put on my warmest clothes and open all the windows and doors—that should cure him!

a 🎧 Listen. You will hear some people talking about problems and possible solutions. What are the solutions?

CONVERSATION	SOLUTIONS	PROBLEMS
1		
2		
3		
4		

📖 Student text page 41

This is the first of three review units. It is designed to consolidate some of the key vocabulary, grammar, and language functions introduced in Units 1–4.

Task 1. (a) Recognizing and matching the same information in different codes is a valuable language learning activity. In this task students try to imagine what the person in each picture is saying and match the picture with the description.
(Answers will vary.)

(b) In pairs, students compare and discuss their choices. Make sure that they are able to give reasons for their choices.

Task 2. (a) In this task students consider both the language structure and what the language is doing—that is, they match the *form* and the *meaning* of the language. Have students do this as an individual writing task.
(Answers: 4—requesting information; 1—expressing disbelief; 3—issuing an invitation; 2—giving advice; 6—responding to an invitation; 5—expressing a preference)

(b) In pairs, students think of situations for each of the conversation extracts. Encourage them to be as specific as they can and to consider the situation—what is happening and who is taking part. Make sure you allow enough time for this part of the task—a minimum of 8 minutes. Then students create their own short dialogues. This part of the task should be allotted a minimum of 10 minutes. (You may choose to allow the discussion to continue for as long as the students are interested and actively involved.) Circulate and correct grammar and content before students use the dialogues for speaking practice.

Task 3. (a)🎧 Play the tape once and have students listen for and write down the possible solutions discussed.
(Answers: 1—take the subway, then the bus; don't ride with someone who's looking for a new job. 2—lock the man out. 3—buy a special birthday card. 4—threw roommate's belongings out of window.)

(b) 🎧 Play the tape a second time and have students listen for and write down the problems that relate to each solution. Have students discuss these problems in small groups. Elicit answers from around the class. (Answers: 1—getting to work; 2—man playing music too loud; 3—what to buy as a birthday present; 4—messy apartment)

(c) In pairs, students consider the problems again. Each student then chooses one of the problems. Each student relates the problem to his or her partner, who gives advice on what to do. Then they switch roles. Circulate and monitor content and pronunciation.

Task 4. **(a)** Write on the board the statement that was overheard. Read it aloud to the class several times. Give students time to think about what the situation might be. Brainstorm their ideas, and write them on the board. Have students work in pairs, and give them time to consider each of the question areas and write out one question for each. Circulate and correct spelling and grammar, and make sure the questions are logical triggers for the presumed answers.

(b) Have each pair of students compare and discuss their questions with another pair. Then, still in pairs, students brainstorm answers to the questions and act them out in a role play. Circulate and monitor pronunciation and grammar.

Task 5. **(a)** One of the most challenging language tasks for students is to create their own language from models and examples that they have been working with. That is what your students will do here. Give them several minutes to consider how they will carry out each of the functions in the list—that is, what exactly they will say.

(b) Have students work in pairs to study the list of requests and decide in what order they might make them if they were talking on the phone to someone at the restaurant.

(c) Have the pairs of students role-play the phone conversation. Make sure that each student plays both parts. Circulate and check content and pronunciation.

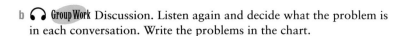

b 🎧 **Group Work** Discussion. Listen again and decide what the problem is in each conversation. Write the problems in the chart.

c **Pair Work** Role play. Choose one of the problems and ask your partner for advice.

Task 4

a **Pair Work** You are at a party and you overhear someone say "I was there for two weeks before they rescued me."

On the blank lines below, write down the questions you would like to ask this person.

Who .... ? When .... ?
What .... ? Where .... ?
Why .... ? How .... ?

b **Group Work** Exchange questions with another pair. Think of answers to their questions and then role play the situation.

Task 5

a Imagine you are talking to someone at the restaurant on the phone. In what order would you make these requests? Number them.

WHAT WOULD YOU SAY?

.... **To make a reservation at a restaurant**
You say: ....
.... **To ask for a table for two**
You say: ....
.... **To find out the address of the restaurant**
You say: ....
.... **To pay by credit card**
You say: ....
.... **To find out what time they open**
You say: ....
.... **To ask for a non-smoking table by the window**
You say: ....

"Could you give me the telephone number of *Le Vent*, please?"

b **Pair Work** Write what you would say on the blank lines above.

c **Pair Work** Role play. Call up and have the conversation. Then change roles and practice again.

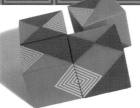

6 That's a Smart Idea

Warm-Up

Unit Goals

In this unit you will:

Describe procedures

"The pictures should be arranged in a certain way."

Report what people say

"Tony asked if he could come over tomorrow."

A Well, that looks like a dog to me.

B A dog? I can't see anything in the picture at all.

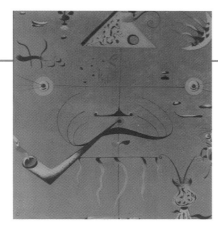

1 This painting is by the famous Catalunyan painter Joan Miró. How many different objects can you see in the picture?

2 GroupWork Discussion. What problems are these inventions designed to solve?

a Floors that are wired so that when somebody drops their clothes, their books, or their toys, a buzzer goes off. If that person doesn't pick up their things in ten seconds, they get an electric shock.

b Telephones that tell teenagers that their 15 minutes are up and to go do their homework, and then disconnects them.

c Televisions that when the channel is changed more than 10 times in 10 minutes, will announce in a deep voice that the person watching should do something useful, like fix the sink. The set will then shut itself off and expel a puff of smoke.

d Alarm clocks that don't ring or play nice music. They squeal and shout threats and automatically back up out of your reach when you try to shut them off.

📖 Student text page 43

Warm-Up

Unit Goals. This section presents the language of describing procedures and reporting what people say. Read out each goal and sample language or have individual students read them. Have students circle the ones that they can do in English.

1. Have students do this task individually. Ask volunteers for responses, and remind them to use the sample language as a model.
(Answers will vary.)

2. With the whole class, read through each of the inventions. Then, in groups, students discuss what problem each invention is designed to solve. It is important to give learners opportunities to voice their opinions and hear those of others, and to speculate from their own knowledge and experience.
(Possible answers: a—messiness; b—excessive phone use; c—excessive channel surfing; d—oversleeping)

Task Chain 1: Creative work

Learning Strategy. Discuss with students the importance of classifying or grouping new information in ways that help them make sense of and remember it.

Task 1. (a) Remind students that words can be grouped in many different ways—words that mean the same or similar things; words that look similar (that is, in shape, length, or spelling); and words about the same topic or subject. In pairs, students group these words under the two headings.
(Answers: "Feeling" Words—creative, holistic, emotional, impulsive, intuitive; "Thinking" Words—analytical, logical, calculating)

(b) Give students time to read through the list of occupations, and make sure that they understand them. Explain, if necessary. Then, in groups, students discuss the qualities important for each of the occupations. Circulate and make sure that students give reasons for their choices. **Variation.** Before the discussion, students read the occupations and write at least two qualities for each one. Then they compare and discuss their choices in groups.
(Answers will vary.)

Task 2. (a) 🎧 Play the tape. In pairs, students listen and fill in the chart. Play the tape again, and have students write down the key words that helped them decide what jobs were likely for Roger and Ingrid.
(Answers will vary.)

(b) Combine two pairs and have students compare and discuss their responses. Make sure that they also give reasons for their responses, using the structure "I think that Roger/Ingrid is a . . . because. . . ."

(c) 🎧 All successful listening involves predicting and then verifying predictions. This task allows students to check the predictions they made in Task 2a. Play the tape again and have students listen to verify their responses.
(Answers: Roger—songwriter; Ingrid—poet)

Task Chain 1 Creative work

my sister

LEARNING STRATEGY
Classifying = putting similar things together in groups.

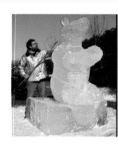

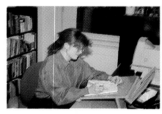

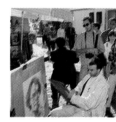

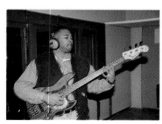

Task 1

a **Pair Work** Classify these words.

creative	logical	emotional	impulsive
analytical	holistic	calculating	intuitive

"Feeling" Words _____   *"Thinking" Words* _____
_____   _____
_____   _____

b **Group Work** Discussion. Which qualities from Task 1a are important for the following occupations? (You can select as many qualities as you want.) Give reasons for your choices.

Occupation	*Qualities*
brain surgeon	_____
composer	_____
politician	_____
editor	_____
other: _____	_____

Task 2

a 🎧 **Pair Work** You will hear two creative people being interviewed about their work. Listen to the first part of the discussion and try to guess what they do. Use the chart to help you. Make a note of the key words that helped you decide.

	PROBABLE		POSSIBLE		IMPROBABLE	
	ROGER	INGRID	ROGER	INGRID	ROGER	INGRID
painter						
poet						
novelist						
musician						
songwriter						
sculptor						

b **Group Work** Compare your responses with another pair and give reasons for your choices.

c 🎧 Now listen to the second part and decide what each person does.

Roger is a _____ .
Ingrid is a _____ .

d 🎧 Listen to the entire interview again. Which of the words from Task 1 can be associated with each person?

Roger ....

Ingrid ....

Task 3

a The following are parts of three employment advertisements. Match the ads and the companies below.

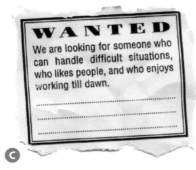

LOOKING for someone who is imaginative, inventive, and loves to be on the move. Must also be able to work late at night.

A

ARE YOU . . . energetic, enthusiastic, talented? We need people like you! Must be prepared to travel.

B

WANTED We are looking for someone who can handle difficult situations, who likes people, and who enjoys working till dawn.

C

.... 1 theater company holding auditions for a national tour

.... 2 discotheque looking for a door person to keep out undesirables

.... 3 a private limousine company looking for drivers for unusual, late-night city tours

b What other qualities would these people need? Complete the ads.

c **Pair Work** Write your own advertisement for one of the following occupations. Exchange it with another pair and guess which occupation the advertisement is for.

computer programmer	dentist	painter
ballet dancer	language teacher	novelist
aerobics instructor	office assistant	architect
taxi driver		

Task 4

a What are the most creative things that you have done in the last:

month? ....

year? ....

b **Group Work** Talk about the things you did.

"Two weeks ago, I made a photo collage for a friend's birthday. Last year, I did a radio program at school with some of my friends."

(d) 🎧 An important listening skill is understanding how information in spoken language is organized. In this task students listen for the words associated with each of the two characters. Elicit answers from around the class.
(Answers: Roger—creative, analytical, logical; Ingrid—creative, holistic, impulsive, intuitive)

Task 3. **(a)** Recognizing and matching the same information in different codes is a valuable language skill. In this reading task students work individually and match the advertisement with the company that placed it. They will need to scan for key clues and information. Elicit responses from around the class.
(Answers: 1—b; 2—c; 3—a)

(b) Have students work in pairs. They discuss other qualities important for doing these jobs successfully.

(c) With the whole class, choose one of the occupations in the list and create a model classified ad on the board. Then, in pairs, students choose another occupation from the list and write their own ad. Make sure they do not put the name of the occupation in the ad. Then combine two pairs to read each other's ad and try to guess the occupation.

Task 4. **(a)** Remind students of the importance of linking the learning to their own lives and opinions. With the whole class, brainstorm possible creative activities that students have done in their studies, in their job, or in their social life. Give students time to think about a specific example either in the past month or in the past year.

(b) Make sure this is a speaking practice task. In small groups, students compare and discuss their creative activities, using the sample language as a model.

Language Focus 1: Passives: past and perfect forms

1. **(a)** Have students complete this task individually. Tell them to be sure to look for key words in the answers.
(Probable answers: 1—I; 2—R; 3—I; 4—I; 5—R)

(b) Have students work in pairs to devise questions that could have inspired these answers. Make sure that the questions and answers go together before students begin to practice them. Remind students that this kind of activity provides opportunities for speaking practice. They should practice the questions and answers line by line so that they can speak from memory rather than having to refer to their books.
(Answers will vary.)

2. Have students work in pairs to try to come up with the right answers. Then have them practice asking and answering the questions, using the sample language as a model.
(Answers will vary—correct answers are not as important here as is practicing the question/answer structure.)

3. **(a)** This task involves students in actively thinking about how English works. Rather than being given the grammar rule, students are encouraged to use examples and models to recognize language patterns and work out grammar/language rules for themselves.
(Answers: 1, 2, 1, 2, 1)

(b) Have students work in pairs to compare answers. Circulate and provide assistance where necessary. With the whole class, work through the list of sentences.

Language Focus 1 Passives: past and perfect forms

1 **a** In Task 2, Roger and Ingrid were asked about the creative process. Who do you think gave these answers? Write "R" for Roger or "I" for Ingrid.

1 .... The key words were written on cards, and the ones that rhymed were put together.
2 .... In most cases the lyrics were written after the tunes.
3 .... I've been asked to get it finished in time for the annual folk festival.
4 .... The lines were written dozens of times.
5 .... It's been recorded by three different groups now.

b **Pair Work** Think of the questions that elicited these answers and practice them. The first one has been done for you.

2 **Pair Work** Trivia quiz. Choose what you think is the correct answer and then practice asking and answering questions.

Australia 1975	Canada 1940	the United States 1993
Brazil 1968	Thailand 1984	the United Kingdom 1989
Japan 1952	Hollywood	

QUESTION	ANSWER
1 When was the Rock Opera *Tommy* composed?	
2 Where was the compact disc invented?	
3 When was the second Woodstock Pop Festival staged?	
4 Where have most of the popular movies been made?	
5 When .... ?	
6 Where .... ?	

3 **a** The passive rather than active voice is used (1) when the action is more important than the person performing the action, and (2) when we don't know who performed the action. Why do you think that the passive was used in the following sentences? Write **1** or **2**.

.... I've been asked to appear on TV to talk about our new show.
.... We had to cancel the show because some of the instruments were stolen.
.... The show was given a great review in yesterday's newspaper.
.... A huge bunch of roses was left at the stage door.
.... The final song was finished a few hours before opening night.

b **Pair Work** Compare your responses with another student.

What's the first thing that happened in writing the poem?

A "Where was *West Side Story* first performed?"

B "I think it was first performed in New York."

Task 1

a **Pair Work** You are about to read a magazine article entitled *Extraordinary Uses for Ordinary Things.* What do you think it will be about? Check [√] one.

☐ Recent inventions for solving everyday household problems
☐ Useful things to do with everyday objects
☐ The year's most extraordinary inventions

b Now read the article on page 48, and write the names of the following items in the appropriate spaces.

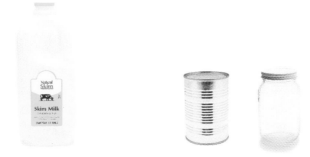

Plastic milk container

A can and a jar

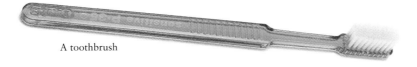

A toothbrush

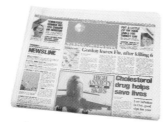

A newspaper

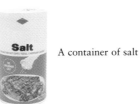

A container of salt

Task Chain 2: I have a great idea!

Task 1. (a) Remind students that predicting is an important part of successful reading. In pairs, students discuss the headline and predict what the article might be about.
(Answer: Useful things to do with everyday objects)

(b) Give students time to read the headings and the paragraphs. Then have them read the paragraphs again and match them with the headings.
(Answers: toothbrush, can/jar, newspaper, salt, milk container)

Task 2. In small groups, students brainstorm extra uses for each of the items in the list. Combine two groups and have them compare and discuss their suggestions.

Task 3. (a) 🎧 Play the tape. Tell students to listen for the problem that is discussed.
(Answer: socks being lost in the washing machine)
   (b) Have students work in small groups to brainstorm possible solutions to the problem. Then combine groups to compare their responses.
   (c) 🎧 Play the tape again. Ask students for the solution, and also ask them for their opinion of Aunt Josephine's idea.
(Answer: attach Velcro to socks so that they won't become separated)
   (d) 🎧 Play the tape once more so that students can listen for the family's objections and then fill in the chart.
(Answers: Danielle—afraid that her skirt would be affected; Todd—afraid of being tangled up in socks and then falling down; Lou—doesn't own matching socks)
   (e) Have students work individually to come up with a similar everyday problem and then brainstorm possible solutions. Ask for responses from around the class. Tell students to use the sample language as a model.

Extraordinary Uses for Ordinary Things

These are too useful to throw away even though they're too worn for their original purpose. Instead use them to:
- clean tiny corners and crevices, such as between bathroom tiles. They're also handy in the car to clean radio knobs and button controls.
- color small sections of your hair accurately.
- scrub away small stains from clothing.

Take the containers to your local recycling center. But what about the lids?
- They make neat saucers for houseplants.
- Small lids can be used as carpet protecters. Place under your furniture legs to prevent marking your carpet.
- The containers themselves can be cleaned and used to store flour, sugar, cookies, pasta, and rice.

- When painting, wet them and apply them to the window panes to keep them clean as you paint the woodwork. Afterwards just peel them off.
- Scrunched up, they are great for cleaning car windows. Wet the windshield, then scrub it down.

- Clean greasy pans by sprinkling a little on and then wiping away with paper.
- A little inside sneakers will absorb odors.

- Great for storing breakfast cereals.
- Ideal as a watering can.
- Make a funnel for pouring oil into the car. Cut the bottom off and turn it upside down.
- Can be used to store soup in the freezer.

Task 2

Group Work Brainstorm. How many additional uses can you think of for the items in the article?

Task 3

a 🎧 Listen to the conversation and identify the problem.

b **Group Work** Brainstorm. How many solutions can you think of for the problem?

c Now listen for Aunt Josephine's solution.

d 🎧 Listen again. Her family objected to the innovative idea. Write their objections in the chart.

"I think that the solution is to buy the black socks."

NAME	OBJECTION
1 Danielle	
2 Todd	
3 Lou	

e Think of a common, everyday problem (like losing one sock). Brainstorm ways of solving the problem, and then identify the pros and cons of each solution.

Language Focus 2 Reported speech

STORY 1

Cousin Danielle said that if the Velcro touched her skirt when she was sitting in class, and the teacher asked her to stand up, it would pull her skirt down. And Uncle Todd said that if he crossed his legs at the ankles, the socks would stick, and when he stood up, he'd fall flat on his face. Cousin Lou said that it wouldn't help him because he didn't have any matching socks anyway!

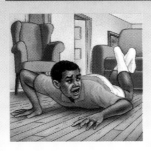

Do you know the rule?

Fill in the chart and compare it with another student. The first one has been done for you.

In reported speech:

this/these	becomes	that/those
here	becomes	....
today/tonight	becomes	....
yesterday	becomes	....
tomorrow	becomes	....
two days ago	becomes	....

1 In Task Chain 2 you heard Josephine's niece tell the story at left. Now figure out the exact words that each person in the story used.

Example
Danielle: "If the velcro touches my skirt when I'm in class and the teacher asks me to stand up, it will pull my skirt down."

Todd: .... Lou: ....

2 Change the following statements into reported speech. Then practice reporting what the people said.

Example
Aunt Josephine: "I can't stand the way this washing machine eats socks."
My aunt said that she couldn't stand the way that washing machine ate socks.

a Aunt Josephine: "I hate the way no one listens to my complaints."
She also said that ....

b Cousin Danielle: "Some people think Mom is eccentric."
My cousin said that ....

c Niece: "I think she's interesting."
I said that ....

d Niece: "She's always had novel solutions to problems."
I also said that ....

3 Look at the following story. Underline the words and phrases that talk about when something happened.

STORY 2

Our English teacher was really mad at everyone the other day. He said that most students had done badly on the exam the day before. He said he'd warned us two days earlier about the exam. Then he said he was going to give us another exam the next day. One of the students asked him not to because there was a concert that night, and most of the students were going. That made the teacher even angrier. He warned us that he was going to give the exam anyway, and told everyone to be there on time.

Language Focus 2: Reported speech

1. Give students time to read the paragraph, which reports what the three people said in the conversation in Task Chain 2. This activity will involve students in actively thinking about how reported speech works in English. Rather than simply being given the rule, students are encouraged to use the examples to figure out the rule for themselves and complete the task.
Optional. If students are having difficulty, you can help by explaining that they will need to change the pronouns to the first person and also change the verbs to the present tense.
(Answers: Todd—"If I cross my legs at the ankles, the socks will stick, and when I stand up, I'll fall flat on my face." Lou—"It won't help me because I don't have any matching socks anyway!")

2. Encourage students to look back at the paragraph and use it as a guide in rewriting the statements as reported speech.
(Answers: a—She also said that she hated the way no one listened to her complaints. b—My cousin said that some people thought Mom was eccentric. c—I said I thought that she was interesting. d—I also said that she'd always had novel solutions to problems.)

Do you know the rule? It is important to give learners opportunities to explain to others what they think or know. In this task students are encouraged to discuss the language patterns they have observed in the previous tasks and their ideas about the rule for using reported speech. Have students do this exercise in pairs.
(Answers: there; yesterday/last night; the day before; the next day; two days before)

3. Have students work individually to read the story and underline the words and phrases denoting when something happened. **Variation.** Do this task as a whole-class exercise.
(Answers: the other day; the day before; two days earlier; the next day; that night)

Self-Check

Communication Challenge

Challenge 6 is on pages 113 and 116 of the student text, and suggestions for its use are on page 113 in this Teacher's Extended Edition.

1. Encourage students to complete this task without looking back at the unit.

2. Students need the opportunity to assess their own progress and make judgments about their own learning. In this task students work individually and rate their performance on the strategies in this unit.

3. Remind students that the You Choose tasks are an important opportunity for them to make some decisions of their own about the learning. Have students prepare the questions before they begin the interview. This will involve deciding how many questions to ask, and what they will be. Students should also make written notes to help them when they are asking the questions. In the interview they should, as much as possible, ask their questions from memory.

4. Have students work individually to check off the words that they know.

• The grammar summary for Unit 6 is on page 131.

Self-Check

COMMUNICATION CHALLENGE

Pair Work Student A: Look at Challenge 6A on page 113. Student B: Look at Challenge 6B on page 116.

HOW WELL DID YOU DO?

1 Write three new sentences or questions you learned.

....

....

....

2 The following are some of the strategies you practiced in this unit. How well can you do these things? Check [√] your answers and then compare with another student.

	Excellent	Good	So-so	Need more practice
• **Selective listening** (listening for the most important words and information)	☐	☐	☐	☐
• **Classifying** (putting similar things together in groups)	☐	☐	☐	☐
• **Making inferences** (using information that is provided to learn new things that are not explicitly stated)	☐	☐	☐	☐

3 **Out of Class** *You choose:* Do **A** or **B**.

A Interview friends and family and make a list of at least three practical problems they have around the home. Bring the list to class and brainstorm possible solutions to the problems.

B Interview three friends or family members about what their "dream" occupation would be. Ask them what personal qualities they think are important for these occupations. Which of these qualities do they think that they possess?

4 Vocabulary check. Check [√] the words you know.

Adjectives/Adverbs

☐ accurately	☐ ideal	☐ probable
☐ analytical	☐ improbable	☐ recycling
☐ calculating	☐ impulsive	☐ smart
☐ emotional	☐ innovative	
☐ employment	☐ intuitive	
☐ everyday	☐ logical	
☐ holistic	☐ possible	

Nouns

☐ aerobics instructor	☐ dentist	☐ sculptor
☐ architect	☐ disco	☐ shock
☐ ballet dancer	☐ event	☐ songwriter
☐ bouncer	☐ musician	☐ taxi driver
☐ buzzer	☐ novelist	☐ Velcro
☐ computer programmer	☐ painter	
	☐ poet	
	☐ procedure	

Verbs

☐ absorb	☐ pour	☐ store
☐ back up	☐ scrub	☐ warn
☐ disconnect	☐ sprinkle	☐ wire

7 Creatures Great and Small

Unit Goals

In this unit you will:

Give definitions

"Mammals are animals that have internal skeletons with backbones."

Express superlatives

"That is the most wonderful sight I have ever seen!"

"I think that the most mysterious creatures live at the bottom of the ocean."

Warm-Up

.... parrot   .... cheetah   .... dog

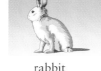 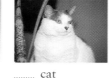

.... dolphin   .... rabbit   .... cat   .... chimpanzee

1 a Group Work Which of these animals make good pets? Which make poor pets? Why? Rank them from best to worst (1 to 7).

b Do you have any pets? What kinds? What do you like or dislike about them?

2 a 🎧 Group Work Trivia quiz. Form teams, then listen to the questions and decide on the answers. Write the letter **A**, **B**, **C**; or **T** for true and **F** for false.

QUESTION	ANSWER
1	
2	
3	
4	
5	
6	

b Now check your answers on page 114.

3 Group Work Discussion.

a What is the most unusual creature you have ever seen?
b What do you think is the most aggressive animal on earth?
c What is the most beautiful insect you have seen?
d Where do the most mysterious creatures live?

📖 Student text page 51

Warm-Up

Unit Goals. This section presents the language of giving definitions and expressing superlatives. Ask individual students to read aloud each of the goals and the examples. Have other students indicate those that they feel they can do in English.

1. (a) Have students work in groups to complete this task. Opinions will vary widely about which animals make the best pets, but the point is for students to practice their speaking skills. Monitor the discussions so that the most talkative students do not dominate. (Answers will vary, but it is obvious that a dog or cat makes a better pet than a dolphin, for example.)

(b) After students think about the questions, call on those students who usually talk less to tell about their experiences and give opinions. If students do not have pets, encourage them to talk about pets that belong to people they know.

2. (a) 🎧 Have students work in groups of at least three to listen to the questions. Play the tape again so that the groups can decide on answers for each question and then fill in the chart.
(Answers: 1—The dodo is (A) an extinct animal. 2—The giant panda is an endangered animal. (T) 3—Kangaroos are considered gourmet food in Australia. (F) 4—Elephants are used as working animals in (A) Thailand. 5—Kiwis are (B) birds. 6—Elderly people who have pets tend to live longer than those who live alone. (T)

(b) In a feedback session with the whole class, check students' answers.

3. Manage this discussion by having students give their opinion and then support it with a reason. **Variation.** Have students read these questions and think about their responses in their own time so that they are prepared for the class discussion.

Task Chain 1: If I could talk with the animals

Learning Strategy.   Point out that we read in different ways, depending on our reason for reading. Skimming is reading for the general idea or gist rather than for the details or specific information.

Task 1.   (a) Read through the list of animals with the whole class and make sure that students know what each animal is. Students then consider the two questions and indicate their answers under the two headings.
(Answers will vary.)
   (b) In pairs, students compare and discuss their answers.

Task 2.   (a) 🎧 An important listening skill is understanding how information in spoken language is organized. In this task students work individually and listen for the animal being talked about. Elicit responses from around the class.
(Answer: a bird)
   (b) 🎧 Play the tape again so that students can identify the topic of the conversation.
(Answer: an animal with incredible communication skills)
   (c) 🎧 Have students work with a partner to compare responses. Then play the tape once more so that students can confirm/revise their answer.

Task 3.   (a) In this task students read the article to get the general feel or gist. Give them time to read the article at least twice. Ask them to mark any words or phrases that help them decide what the reviewer's opinion is. Elicit answers from around the class. Make sure that students give examples from the text to support their answer.
(Answer: Yes, the reviewer liked the program.)
   (b) Have students work in pairs to check their responses.
   (c) Before the discussion, give students time to think about specific instances of animal communication, from their own experiences or those of people

(Continued on page 53.)

Task Chain 1 If I could talk with the animals

LEARNING STRATEGY

Skimming = reading quickly to get a general idea of text.

Task 1

a How well do these animals communicate with each other? Check [√] column A. How well do they communicate with humans? Check [√] column B.

	A COMMUNICATE WITH EACH OTHER			B COMMUNICATE WITH HUMANS		
	Well	**OK**	**Not well**	**Well**	**OK**	**Not well**
dog						
dolphin						
chimpanzee						
parrot						
cat						
rabbit						
cheetah						

b Compare your responses with another student.

Task 2

a 🎧 Listen to the conversation and identify the animal the people are talking about.

b 🎧 Listen again. What is the topic of the conversation?

c **Pair Work** 🎧 Compare responses, then listen once more to confirm your choices.

Task 3

a Skim this review of a television program and decide if the reviewer liked the program.

b **Pair Work** Compare responses with a classmate and give reasons for your choices.

c **Group Work** Discussion. Do you believe that animals have language? How convincing do you find the evidence discussed in the article?

Animal Talk

Interest in the issue of animal communication is on the increase, if the current offerings on television are anything to go by. In the last week, there have been no fewer than five programs dealing with the subject. The most interesting of these was a program aired late last night on TVPM. The programing executives obviously had little idea of the quality of the program, nor of the interest it would generate. It should have been aired in prime time.

The program provided a general look at the issue of animal communication, the basic question being: Do animals have language in the same way as humans have language? However, the show was quickly stolen by an African gray parrot named Nigel. We have all heard parrots talk, but do they have *language?* If we believe what this program showed, the answer must surely be a resounding "yes". Nigel is able to name wooden objects and toys that are pointed out by Irene Pepperberg, the woman who trained him. He can name different types of fruit in the same way.

Most remarkable of all, Nigel is able to communicate his feelings. On one occasion, after he gave a wrong answer, he lowered his head and apologized. Of course, the skeptics would say he has only learned these words as a collection of sounds, but those of us out here in TV land were delighted.

What made the show so delightful was the fact that the producers let Nigel tell his own story. There was no serious professor-type in the background telling us what to think on the issue of animal communication. This is what television is all about—letting words and pictures tell their own story without the interference of "experts." We don't need them to tell us what is obvious to our own eyes. ∎

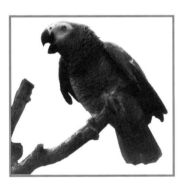

Task 4

a The following notes were made by two speakers preparing for a debate. The topic: Animals can communicate with humans in a meaningful way. Write **F** for *for* or **A** for *against* in the blank before each point to show whether or not it supports the statement.

.... Follow complex commands.
.... Fetch the newspaper on command.
.... Are not conscious of what they're saying.
.... Have no thought behind their actions—process of habit formation.
.... Require long period of training—complex actions broken down into sequence of simple ones.
.... Speak with their owners.

b Now match the opposing statements.

FOR	AGAINST
1	1
2	2
3	3

c GroupWork Debate. Choose three speakers to speak in favor of, and three speakers to speak against the idea that animals can communicate meaningfully with humans. Each speaker speaks for two minutes, and the class then votes on which side presented the most convincing case.

they know. Encourage them to then generalize about animal communication. **Variation.** Have students extend the discussion to consider the difference between factual evidence and the personal opinion of an observer such as the reviewer.

Task 4. **(a)** Write the topic of the debate on the board, and make sure that all students understand it. Working individually, students divide the statements into those that support the argument and those that oppose it.
(Answers: F, F, A, A, A, F)

(b) Students now match each statement with its opposite.
(Answers: 1. Follow complex commands./Require long period of training—complex actions broken down into sequence of simple ones. 2. Fetch the newspaper on command./Have no thought behind their actions—process of habit formation. 3. Speak with their owners./Are not conscious of what they're saying.)

(c) Have two teams of students debate the subject of animal communication. Each team consists of three volunteers. Divide the rest of the class into two groups, and have each group help one of the teams. These students decide which main point will be made by each speaker and any supplementary or supporting points that must be considered.

Encourage the debaters to think of real-life examples to support their stand. Explain to the class that formal debating differs from conversational discussion or argument. In the debate, each speaker has a maximum of two minutes, *uninterrupted,* to state his or her position. **Optional.** Form new teams and repeat the process.

Language Focus 1: Relative clauses
with *that* and *whose*

1. **(a)** In pairs, students practice saying the statements. One student says the first part, and the other completes it with one of the possible endings. Explain that there is more than one correct answer for some of the statements. Circulate and check content and pronunciation.
(Answers will vary but should be plausible.)
   (b) Students swap roles and practice the statements again.

2. **(a)** Have students do this task individually. It will work as either a speaking task or a writing task.
(Answers: 1—Dinosaurs were reptiles that ruled the earth for 160 million years. 2—Snakes are cold-blooded animals that live on land and in water. 3—Vertebrates are animals that have a skeleton and a backbone. 4—Whales are mammals that live in water. 5—Bats are vertebrates that can fly.)
   (b) With the whole class, create the beginnings of definitions or describing statements using *that*. The statements could be about animals, but they could also be about other subjects—for example, "English is a language that. . . ."

3. Have students do this task individually. Circulate and check responses.
(Answers: a—Seals are water-dwelling mammals whose offspring are born on land. b—Mammals are animals whose young are fed on milk. c—Emus are birds whose wings are too short to enable them to fly. d—Snakes are reptiles whose skin is shed each year.

4. **(a)** Divide the class into groups of at least five so that each students can contribute one question to the quiz. Circulate and correct the questions. **Variation.** Each group decides on a subject area for its questions—for example, animals, humans, plants, natural phenomena, manufactured objects.

(Continued on page 55.)

Language Focus 1 Relative clauses with *that* and *whose*

A Reptiles are animals that . . .

B . . .have cold blood.

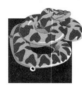

A This animal is a reptile that is now extinct.

B A dinosaur!

1 a Pair Work Student A: Say the first part of the statement. Student B: Complete the statement.

Student A	Student B
1 Reptiles are animals that . . .	feed their young milk.
2 Insects are animals that . . .	have warm blood.
3 Mammals are animals that . . .	are covered with feathers.
4 Birds are animals that . . .	live in water.
5 Fish are animals that . . .	eat flesh.
	have cold blood.
	have six legs.
	can fly.
	lay eggs.

b Pair Work Now change roles and do the task again.

2 a Combine these sentences following. The first one has been done for you.

   Example: Mammals are animals. Mammals have warm blood.
   "Mammals are animals that have warm blood."

   1 Dinosaurs were reptiles. Dinosaurs ruled the earth for 160 million years.
   2 Snakes are cold-blooded animals. Snakes live on land and in water.
   3 Vertebrates are animals. They have a skeleton and a backbone.
   4 Whales are mammals. Whales live in water.
   5 Bats are vertebrates. They can fly.

b Pair Work Practice making statements using *that*.

3 Combine these sentences following the example.

   Example: Mammals are animals. Their offspring have warm blood.
   "Mammals are animals whose offspring have warm blood."

   a Seals are water-dwelling mammals. Their offspring are born on land.
   b Mammals are animals. Their young are fed on milk.
   c Emus are birds. Their wings are too short to enable them to fly.
   d Snakes are reptiles. Their skin is shed each year.

4 a Group Work Make up your own trivia quiz. Think of five descriptions like the one at left.

b Group Work Now compete with another group. Take turns asking and answering each other's trivia questions.

Task Chain 2 Into the wild

Task 1

a Check [√] the words you know.

☐ interesting   ☐ precious   ☐ beautiful
☐ magical   ☐ wonderful   ☐ exciting
☐ dramatic   ☐ incredible   ☐ difficult
☐ endangered

b **PairWork** Compare responses with a partner.

c Which words could be used to describe the creatures in these pictures?

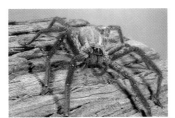
A hunting spider

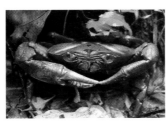
A land crab

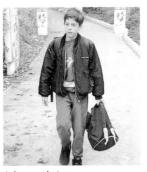
A human being

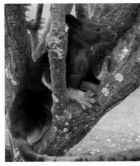
A tree kangaroo

Task 2

a 🎧 Listen to the inteview and circle the words in Task 1a that you hear.

b What does the naturalist say about these creatures?

hunting spider: ....
land crabs: ....
tree kangaroo: ....
human beings: ....

(b) Combine two groups, and have them ask and answer each other's quiz questions. Encourage students to ask the questions from memory if possible. Circulate and correct pronunciation.

Task Chain 2: Into the wild

Task 1. **(a)** Have students work individually to mark off the words that they know. Remind students that grouping words is a good vocabulary learning strategy. You may group words together because they mean the same or similar things, because they look alike (in shape, length, or spelling), or because they are linked to the same topic or subject. **Variation.** In pairs, students group the words in some way—for example, choosing the words that do not have three syllables *(precious, incredible)*.

(b) Students compare their list with a partner.

(c) Have students work individually to give their responses, and then ask for volunteers to explain why they chose the words that they did. This will allow students to compare their own perspectives with those of others in the class.

Task 2. **(a)** 🎧 Play the tape. Working individually, students listen for any of the words listed in Task 1a. (Answers: all the words except *wonderful*)

(b) Play the tape again and have students write what the naturalist says about each of the creatures listed. Elicit answers from around the class. (Answers: hunting spider—dramatic; land crabs—incredible; tree kangaroo—endangered; human beings—uninteresting)

Task 3. Remind students of the reading strategy of scanning—that is, not reading every word, but reading to find specific information. Have students scan the letters and note any points for or points against the protection of the tree kangaroo.
(Answers will vary but should be supported by the letters.)

Task 4. (a) Have each student select the letter that he or she disagrees with. Have students make notes on what they will say in the letter and write a first/rough draft. Circulate and correct spelling and grammar. Then have students write a second draft incorporating your corrections.

(b) Students work in pairs with another student who has expressed a different point of view. They read each other's letter and discuss their differences of opinion.

Task 3

These letters to the editor appeared in an Australian newspaper. Read the letters and note the points in favor of and the points against the protection of the tree kangaroo.

Dear Editor,

I read with disgust your article on the tree kangaroo. According to your article, the tree kangaroo is faced with extinction because of the destruction of its native habitat by "evil" logging companies. Well, I am the chief executive officer of the largest logging company in the Tatawangalo State Forest region, and I strongly disagree with some of the points that your reporter made.

Your article asserts that the tree kangaroo is an endangered species. This is untrue. I have seen three of these creatures in the last three weeks. My workers also report frequent sightings of the kangaroo.

Even if the tree kangaroo is in danger of extinction, this is not a good reason to stop cutting down trees. Species have been dying out ever since the planet first began to evolve. It's a natural process. When was the last time that you saw a dinosaur? The planet has been getting along quite nicely without these creatures for millions of years.

If logging were to be stopped, it would mean the extinction of loggers, who, in my view, are far more important than kangaroos. In my opinion, there is something seriously wrong with individuals who put animals before humans. And it's not just the loggers and their families who would suffer. We would all suffer. The economy, which is in pretty poor shape at the moment, depends heavily on the export of natural products such as our forest timbers.

In the future, you should think carefully before printing such a one-sided article.

Yours,
Humans Have Rights, Too, You Know

Dear Editor,

I was dismayed by the article in your newspaper on the possibility of the extinction of the tree kangaroo. Two years ago, I took my family on a camping holiday in the Tatawangalo State Forest. It is one of the happiest holidays that we've ever had—in one of the most beautiful places on earth. The only thing that shattered our peace was the constant noise of the loggers destroying the natural beauty of the place with their chain saws. While we were in the forest, we saw several of the delightful but very shy tree kangaroos. This was definitely the high point of the trip for my children. It fills me with sorrow and shame to think that *their* children might never have the chance to see these lovely creatures in their native habitat. People just don't seem to realize that once something is extinct it is lost forever.

I would like to close by thanking you for your article, and for making the public aware of the endangered tree kangaroo.

Sincerely,
Nature Lover

Task 4

a Select the letter you disagree with, and write a response. Summarize the points made in the letter, then state your objections to these, and give reasons.

b Exchange letters with a student who has expressed a different point of view from you, then discuss your differences of opinion.

Dear Humans Have Rights Too,

In your letter to the editor, you state that ...
....
....

I believe that you are wrong for the following reasons:
....
....

Sincerely,

Language Focus 2 Superlative adjectives with present perfect

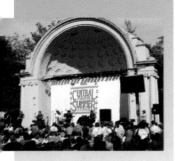

Do you know the rule?

a **PairWork** Look back over the unit and make a list of adjectives that can fill the pattern:
What's the most (*adjective*) (*noun*) you've ever (*verb*)?

b When do we use *most + adjective* and when do we use *adjective + -est*?

"What's the most interesting thing you've ever done?"

"The most adventurous trip Tomoko has ever taken was a shopping trip to Macy's!"

"The most annoying thing that happened to us was being delayed at the airport before we left for Seoul."

---

1 **PairWork** Match these questions and answers and then practice them with a partner.

Questions
a What's the most interesting thing you've ever done, Tom?
b What's the most beautiful sight you've ever seen, Sally?
c When's the best time to visit Thailand?
d What's the greatest experience Sam and Nadia have ever had?
e What's the most adventurous trip they've ever taken?
f Who's the most unusual person you've ever met?
g Why did you say that going to Mexico was the best vacation you've ever taken?

Answers
.... Going to a rock concert in Central Park.
.... A boat trip up the Amazon.
.... The culture, the food, the people, the climate, and the sights were perfect.
.... The guy who wrote the rock opera *Tommy*.
.... Learning how to paint.
.... I guess December, because it's not too hot.
.... Seeing the sun set over Manhattan from the top of Rockefeller Center.

2 a **PairWork** Discussion. Ask and answer questions with your partner about the . . .

- most interesting thing they've ever done
- hardest thing they've ever done
- most beautiful sight they've ever seen
- most incredible experience they've ever had
- oldest movie they've ever seen
- most adventurous trip they've ever taken
- most unusual person they've ever met

b **GroupWork** Tell another pair about your partner's experiences.

3 a **PairWork** Discuss the following things that happened to you on a journey or vacation.

- the most interesting/unusual thing
- the best thing
- the most frightening thing
- the most unpleasant/worst thing
- the most annoying thing

b **GroupWork** Tell another pair about your experiences.

Language Focus 2: Superlative adjectives with present perfect

---

1. Go through the list of questions with the whole class. Prompt students by using the key phrase from each sentence—for example, *most interesting thing; best vacation*. Allow time for students to choose answers from the list below.
(Answers: a—learning how to paint; b—Manhattan sunset; c—December; d—rock concert; e—Amazon boat trip; f—*Tommy*'s writer; g—the culture, the food, etc.)

Do you know the rule? It is important to give learners opportunities to explain to others what they think or know. In this task students are encouraged to discuss the language patterns that they have observed in the previous tasks and their ideas about the rule for using reported speech. Have students do this activity in pairs.
(Answers will vary.)

2. (a) Allow students to make notes if they wish. Then they work in pairs to practice asking and answering the questions. Circulate and make sure this is a speaking practice task. Correct content and pronunciation as needed.
(b) Combine two pairs and have each student tell the group about his or her partner, using the sample language as a guide.

3. (a) Learning is more successful when learning tasks have a specific focus. Give students time to think about at least three specific journeys or vacations that fit one or more of the descriptions in the list. These could have happened in the recent past or many years ago. Then, in pairs, students compare and discuss their stories.
(b) Have each pair of students share responses with another pair.

Self-Check

Communication Challenge

Challenge 7 is on pages 115 and 117 of the student text, and suggestions for its use are on page 115 in this Teacher's Extended Edition.

1. Encourage students to complete this task without looking back at the unit.

2. (a) In this task students work individually and rate their performance on the strategies they have practiced in this unit. Then, in pairs, they compare and discuss their progress.
    (b) In groups of at least three, students brainstorm ideas about which of these strategies they would use outside the classroom and where and why they would use them. Circulate and make sure the suggestions are as specific as possible. Encourage students to think about situations they have been in when they needed to use these strategies.

3. An important strategy in language learning is finding out more about what we need or want to know. Encourage students to collect information in different ways—for example, by asking travel agency personnel for information and by collecting and reading written information.

4. Have students work individually to check off the words that they know.

*   The grammar summary for this unit is on page 131.

Self-Check

COMMUNICATION CHALLENGE

Pair Work Student A: Look at Challenge 7A on page 115. Student B: Look at Challenge 7B on page 117.

1 Write three new sentences or questions you learned.

....

....

....

2 a Pair Work Here are some of the strategies you practiced in this unit. How well can you do these things? Check [√] your answers and then compare with another student.

HOW WELL DID YOU DO?

	Excellent	Good	So-so	Need more practice
Role playing (pretending to someone else and using the right language for the situation you are in)	☐	☐	☐	☐
Skimming (reading quickly to get a general idea of a text)	☐	☐	☐	☐
Choosing (selecting the task you want to do from two alternatives)	☐	☐	☐	☐

b Group Work Brainstorm. Which of these strategies would you use out of class? Where? For what purposes?

3 Out of Class Visit a travel agency and collect information and any brochures in English describing interesting and unusual tours. Bring them to class and talk about them.

4 Vocabulary check. Check [√] the words you know.

Adjectives/Adverbs

☐ adventurous	☐ extinct	☐ remarkable
☐ aggressive	☐ extreme	☐ seriously
☐ complex	☐ magical	☐ shy
☐ convincing	☐ meaningfully	☐ surely
☐ delightful	☐ opposing	☐ unpleasant
☐ endangered	☐ precious	☐ wonderful

Nouns

☐ chimpanzee	☐ extinction	☐ mammal
☐ crab	☐ feelings	☐ offspring
☐ creature	☐ habitat	☐ parrot
☐ definition	☐ habit- formation	☐ reptile
☐ destruction		☐ sequence
☐ dinosaur	☐ insect	☐ skeptic
☐ disgust	☐ interest	☐ spider
☐ dolphin	☐ interference	☐ vertebrate
☐ eco-trip	☐ kangaroo	☐ whale

Verbs

☐ air	☐ name	☐ shed
☐ apologize	☐ rule	☐ skim
☐ communicate	☐ shatter	

8 Communications

Warm-Up

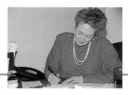

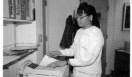 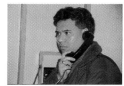 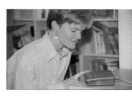

Unit Goals

In this unit you will:

Describe intentions

"I plan to give up trying to communicate with my neighbor—he's impossible."

Make indirect requests

"I wonder if you could help us design a new logo."

1 What methods of communication are these people using?

2 **a** Pair Work Think of several ways of completing the following statements.

"I find it really difficult communicating in the following situations:"

....

"I enjoy communicating in the following situations:"

....

b Group Work What makes communication easy? Difficult?

3 **a** Do you know English expressions for the following situations?

1 showing that you don't understand
2 checking that you have understood the other person
3 checking that the other person has correctly understood you

b What are these people doing? Match each statement to a situation from Task 3a. Put the correct number in the blank.

1 .... "Did you say she won a million bucks?"
2 .... "Excuse me?"
3 .... "Then you take a left off 21st Street. You know where I mean?"

LEARNING STRATEGY

Memorizing conversational patterns and expressions = learning phrases to start conversations and keep them going.

📖 Student text page 59

Warm-Up

Unit Goals. This section presents the language of describing intentions and making indirect requests. Choose individual students to read out each of the goals and the examples. Ask students which goals they think they can do in English.

1. Have students do this task individually. **Optional.** Have them work in pairs to compare and discuss their responses. In either case, elicit answers from around the class.
(Answers: top photo—writing a letter; bottom left photo—sending a fax; bottom center photo—making a phone call; bottom right photo—using an answering machine)

2. (a) With the whole class, read through each of the statements. Then have pairs of students discuss different ways to complete the statements. Circulate and correct content, spelling, and grammar.
  (b) Do this task as a whole-class discussion. You may wish to guide the discussion so that there is also a focus not only on what students say but also on how they say it. **Variation.** Have students discuss whether there are communication situations that they enjoy or find difficult in English but that they do not enjoy or find difficult in their first language.

3. (a) Have students work individually to provide responses. Check answers from around the class.
  (b) Students match the questions to the situations in 3a.
(Answers: Question 1—2; Question 2—1; Question 3—3)

Learning Strategy. Stress the importance of looking for and memorizing patterns and expressions in conversations. Learning "set phrases" or expressions is an important part of learning a new language.

Task Chain 1: Can I put you on hold?

Task 1. (a) Remind students that surveys are not only a way of gathering information; in the classroom, surveys are a good way to help learners find out more about one another and also a good way to create a friendly and supportive learning environment. Give students time to read the list, and make sure that they understand the communications devices. Explain, if necessary. Then have students check off the ones that they use before filling in the rest of the chart.

(b) In groups of at least three, students compare their responses, using the sample language structure, and then discuss any differences. Make sure that this is a speaking practice task.

Task 2. (a) Make this an individual reading task. Give students time to read the headings and then read through each of the extracts. Ask students to mark the words or phrases in each extract that helped them choose the heading for it. Elicit answers from around the class.
(Answers: Call Waiting; Speed Calling; Three-Way Calling; Call Forwarding; Caller ID)

Task Chain 1 Can I put you on hold?

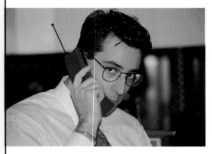

"Last week I called my ex-girlfriend and left an invitation to lunch on her voice mail. But she never called back."

Task 1

a Survey. The following are all ways of communicating over a phone line. Check [√] the ones you use. For the devices you use write down how often you use them (twice a week, once a month, etc.). When was the last time you used each? Who did you communicate with? What did you communicate about? Fill in the chart.

	HOW OFTEN	WHEN	TO WHOM	ABOUT
☐ regular telephone				
☐ mobile telephone				
☐ answering machine				
☐ fax				
☐ voice mail				

b Group Work Compare your responses with three or four other students' responses.

Task 2

a Look at this page from the front of a telephone directory. Match the headings with the customer calling services described below.

Three-Way Calling   **Speed Calling**   **Call Waiting**
Call Forwarding   **Caller ID**

Customer Calling Services

These optional calling services are available in all of the exchanges in this directory to one-party service customers only.

■ ....
When you're on the phone, a beep tone lets you know if another person is calling you. The person calling you hears only the normal ringing. You can then put the first caller on hold and talk to the second caller.

■ ....
Lets you program your phone to dial frequently called local or long distance numbers by using just one or two digits.

■ ....
Lets you add a third person to your conversation whether or not you have received or placed the first call.

■ ....
Lets you transfer your incoming calls to another telephone number.

■ ....
Tells you the number of the person calling when your phone rings.

b **Which telephone services would you recommend for the following people? (Some may need more than one service.)**

1 Your sister runs a telephone dating service. People call her up, and she puts them in touch with other callers by phone.

2 Your brother runs a small direct-mail business from home. The warehouse that dispatches his products for him is often busy, and he wastes a lot of time trying to get through to them. He also has a lot of incoming and outgoing calls.

3 Your neighbor runs a window-cleaning service. He is out on the road most of the day.

4 Your elderly aunt is confined to her home. Her only means of communicating is through the telephone, which she finds difficult because she has arthritis (a disease of the joints) in her hands.

c **PairWork** Compare answers and give reasons for your choices.

d **GroupWork** Discussion. Which of these services would you like? Rank them from most to least useful (1–5). Give reasons.

Task 3

a 🎧 Listen to the three conversations and decide which of the Customer Calling Services is being used in each case.

CONVERSATION	CUSTOMER CALLING SERVICE
1	
2	
3	

b 🎧 **PairWork** Compare responses with another student and then listen again to check your answers.

Task 4

You choose: Do Ⓐ or Ⓑ.

Ⓐ a **PairWork** You and your partner are going into business together. Decide what kind of business you are starting, and then decide which of the telephone services from Task 2 you would like to have.

Ⓑ a Select one of the calling services from Task 2, and think of reasons why the service is valuable.

b **PairWork** You are a telephone company sales representative. Try to convince your partner to get the calling service you selected.

(b) With the whole class, read through the descriptions, or choose individual students to read them. Then, working individually, students choose a telephone service that would meet each person's needs. Circulate and provide assistance where necessary. (Possible answers: 1—Call Forwarding, Call Waiting; 2—Speed Calling, Call Waiting; 3—Call Forwarding; 4—Speed Calling)

(c) In pairs, students compare their responses and give reasons for them. Giving and supporting opinions, and speculating from experience and knowledge are important in developing language skills. This task gives students a chance to practice these skills.

(d) Before the discussion, have each student consider which of the services he or she would find most useful and rank them accordingly. Then students compare and discuss their views in groups.

Task 3. (a) 🎧 Play the tape, pausing after each conversation to allow students to make notes. Play the tape again so that students can check their notes and fill in their answers.
(Answers: 1—Call Forwarding; 2—Three-Way Calling; 3—Call Waiting)

(b) 🎧 In pairs, students compare and discuss their answers. Then play the tape again and have them confirm their responses.

Task 4. A. Tell students doing this task to be very specific about who the participants are, what the conversation is about, and what the request is. Then, in pairs, they role-play their conversation while another pair listens and then tries to guess the situation and the service. Then have the pairs switch roles.

B. (a) Students choose one of the telephone services. Then they think of specific situations and discuss reasons people might have for using this service. Encourage them to be as specific as possible.

(b) Have students work in pairs. One student is the phone company's sales representative, who tries to sell the other student on the idea of the service chosen in (a).

Language Focus 1: Two-part verbs + gerunds

1. In this task students are encouraged to read the sentences carefully and guess word meaning from context. Have them work individually. Circulate and provide assistance as necessary. With the whole class, go through the list and check responses.
(Answers: a—continue; b—stop; c—postponed; d—tolerate)

2. (a) Give students time to read the extract at least twice. Then have them fill in the blanks with the appropriate verbs.
(Answers: keep on; looks forward to; giving up)
(b) Have students work in pairs to compare and discuss their responses.

3. (a) Have students work individually to provide appropriate responses.
(Suggested answers: 1—I have. I'm looking forward to it. 2—It was. We're cutting down on calls. 3—No, he/she couldn't go through with it. 4—I did. I'm planning on playing this afternoon.)
(b) Circulate and make sure all answers are plausible before students begin practicing them with a partner. Have all students practice both asking and answering.

4. (a) Remind students of the importance of linking the learning to their own lives and opinions. Guide them to think about specific situations and plans or intentions they have. Make this an individual writing task. Circulate and correct spelling and grammar.
(b) Have students work in pairs. Remind them that this task is designed to give them the chance to practice their speaking.

Language Focus 1 Two-part verbs + gerunds

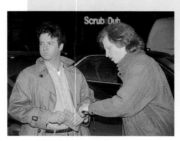

1 Rewrite the following sentences. Replace each underlined two- or three-part verb with one of these verbs: *postpone, tolerate, stop, continue.*

a I'm not going to <u>keep on</u> calling someone who never calls back.
b Steve says that he's going to <u>give up</u> trying to fax the West Coast office. He can never get through.
c I've <u>put off</u> calling Sally because I'll have to tell her she didn't get the promotion she was after.
d We're moving because we can't <u>put up with</u> those noisy neighbors.

2 a Fill in the blanks with the appropriate two-part verbs.

keep on   **giving up**   **looks forward to**

When faced with a difficult communication situation, different people react in different ways. Some people .... talking as though nothing unusual had happened. Others avoid conflict whenever it occurs. Occasionally you meet someone who .... participating in difficult situations, seeing these as a challenge. A few people deal with the situation by .... communicating completely.

b **Pair Work** Check your responses with another student's responses.

3 a Think of an appropriate response to the following statements and questions using the verb in parentheses.
Example: "I thought you were going to stop smoking this year?"
          (give up) "I am. I give up smoking every year."

1 I hear you've finally accepted that new job.
  (look forward to) ....
2 Our phone bill was huge this month.
  (cut down on) ....
3 Did the boss fire that incompetent worker yet?
  (not go through with) ....
4 I see that you booked a court at the tennis club.
  (take up) ....

b **Pair Work** Now practice them with another student.

4 a Think of plans and intentions you have and complete these statements.
1 I plan to keep on ....
2 I think I'll cut down on ....
3 I'm not going to put off ....
4 I think I'll take up ....
5 I plan on ....

b **Pair Work** Now practice the statements with a partner.

Task Chain 2 Image makers!

"Well, a logo says a lot about a company. So does the slogan that they use."

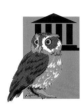

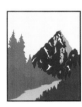

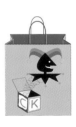

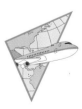

Task 1

a What is a "logo?" Find the derivation of the word in your dictionary.

b **Pair Work** Look at these logos. What "message" does each convey? Make a list of several words to describe each logo.

c **Group Work** Compare your list with another pair. Discuss what kinds of companies these logos might belong to.

Task 2

Group Work In the next task you will listen to a communications consultant talking about his work with large corporations. Discuss the ways in which corporations and other organizations communicate information about themselves.

Task 3

a 🎧 Listen to the tape and identify the two corporations being discussed, the problem each one had, and the solution.

CORPORATION	PROBLEM	SOLUTION
1		
2		

b 🎧 **Pair Work** Listen again and find the logos for the corporations that are mentioned.

Task 4

a **Group Work** Role play. Select one of the following scenarios and brainstorm solutions for the problem. Try to think of as many different solutions as you can, and then decide on the best one.

Scenario 1: You work for a company that is trying to break into a market in another country. The company has a strong public image—an image closely associated with the logo, company slogan, and advertising campaign. Unfortunately, your logo has negative connotations in the new country. If you keep the logo, slogan, and advertisements, it is unlikely that the product will be accepted in this new country. If you change them, your corporate image will suffer at home and elsewhere abroad.

Scenario 2: You work for a company that produces luxury motor vehicles. Several of the vehicles have been found to have faulty braking systems. All the vehicles should be recalled for inspection. However, the company is afraid to place advertisements in the media calling for the return of the cars because its image will suffer.

Task Chain 2: Image makers!

Task 1. (a) Students look up the word *logo* in their dictionaries. Have them look for both meaning and derivation. Then, with the whole class, discuss the range of meanings found.

(b) There are many ways of interpreting the messages in the logos, so this task gives students the chance to bring their own personal views to the learning. Give students time to study the logos individually before they discuss their ideas with a partner.

(c) Combine two pairs and have students compare and discuss their ideas.

Task 2. Do this task with the whole class, and organize the discussion into three clear stages. First, have students brainstorm the names of large (real-life) corporations. Second, what are some of the things that students know about these companies? Third, how did students get this knowledge—from radio, television, magazines, brochures, advertisements?

Task 3. (a) 🎧 Play the tape three times, once for each of the stages of the task, and have students take notes. The first time students listen for the names of the two corporations; the second time they listen for the problem each corporation had; the third time they listen for the solution to each of the problems. (Answers: 1—West-East Banking Corporation; trouble entering Asian markets because of faulty logo; developed new logo. 2—Deep Springs; impurities found in bottles; admission of problem to journalists)

(b) 🎧 Have students work in pairs. Play the tape again so that students can match each corporation with its logo. (Answers: West-East—owl; Deep Springs—mountain)

Task 4. (a) With the whole class, read through each scenario and make sure that all students understand them. In small groups, students then choose one of the problems listed and brainstorm solutions for it. Combine two groups and have them compare and discuss their suggestions and decide on the best one.

(Continued on page 64.)

(b) Reorganize the class so that each group works with a group that has discussed a different problem. Stress to students that the objective of the discussion is to share ideas and opinions, not to arrive at consensus.

Task 5. **(a)** With the whole class, choose words from the first advertisement that suggest a product or service being advertised. Then, working in pairs, students do this for the second advertisement and choose words that could fill the gaps.
(Answers will vary.)

(b) Put two pairs together to compare and discuss their ideas. As much as possible, make this a speaking practice task, with students using the sample language as a model.

(c) It is important for learners to have the chance to give their own opinions, to hear those of others, and to speculate from the combined knowledge and experience. In groups, students share their opinions on why companies advertise the way they do, and discuss the kind of language companies use to create their image and appeal to the public.
(Answers will vary.)

Scenario 3: You work for a company that manufactures clothing. Due to increased competition, sales have fallen, and the company has laid off some of its workers. This has led to a general drop in morale, which is further damaging the ability of your company to compete. If you could guarantee workers there will be no more lay-offs, morale would increase. However, while you hope that there will be no more lay-offs, you cannot guarantee this.

b **Group Work** Compare your solutions with the solutions of a group that has worked on a different problem. Discuss the different types of solutions.

Task 5

a **Pair Work** Most of the identifying words have been removed from these advertisements. Make a list of the things that each ad might be used for to sell. Can you guess any of the words that have been removed?

"Well, the first one might be used to sell soap, health food, deodorant, skin cream, or even mineral water."

> A simple and straight-forward .... and fitness line created by .... for today's active, health-focused lifestyles. These are no-nonsense, nutrient-based products that protect and condition your .... Like a .... with .... Or an all-over .... and body .... that's sweat-resistant, water resistant, and fortified with .... Plus a .... to keep you .... and .... Pure. Basic. Easy.

> It's not for everyone. But isn't that the beauty of it? It's one thing to be wanted by all. It's quite another to be obtainable by only a few. The .... is decidedly the latter. With a bias towards luxury, the .... is a study in elegance. It abounds with refinements, from the .... to the .... on the .... and .... Its .... give it the responsive agility you demand of a .... And it has the .... features .... you would expect from a .... of this caliber. Which can be a beautiful thing in itself. Some things are worth the price.

b **Group Work** Compare your responses with another pair, then comment on each other's ideas.

c **Group Work** Discussion. The companies in Task 5a have tried to create a distinctive corporate image through their advertisements. What kind of image are the ads trying to promote (quality, value, environmentally-friendly, etc.)? Which words and phrases are used to achieve this? What age group are the ads aimed at? What social group? Which image appeals to you?

Language Focus 2 Indirect questions & requests

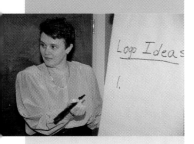

1 Change these direct requests into indirect questions.

Example:
"I wonder if you could help us to design a new corporate logo?"
"Could you help us to design a new corporate logo?"

a Can you let us know how expensive it will be?

....

b Do you think it will make a difference to our image?

....

c When do you think you could have it done?

....

d What do you imagine the problem with our image is?

....

e Do you know if the new logo is ready?

....

2 **Pair Work** Now practice them with a partner.

3 **Pair Work** One student takes the A role and the other takes the B role.

Student A
a Add three items to the following hypothetical situations, and then use them to make requests.

   1 Your apartment is being painted and you have to get out for a few days.
   2 Your family is visiting and you have no room for them in your apartment.
   3 You need to pay a large bill, but are temporarily out of money.
   4 ....
   5 ....
   6 ....

b Now change roles and do the task again.

Student B
a Your partner is going to make a number of unusual requests. Reply to each request.
b Now use your own three additional items and change roles.

4 a Write several requests that you would like another student to make.

b **Pair Work** Exchange requests with another student and go around the class and make the requests.

"I wonder if I could move in with you for a few days?"

"I'm sorry, my parents are here for the weekend."

"Would you ask Yumiko if she could bring her book on Zen to school tomorrow?"

A Yumiko, can you bring your book on Zen to school for Alan tomorrow?

B Unfortunately, I don't have it any more—I left it on the bus last week.

Language Focus 2: Indirect questions and requests

1. Rather than being given the rule for indirect questions and requests, students are encouraged to use the example to figure out the rule for themselves and then complete the task.
(Suggested answers: a—I wonder if you can tell me how expensive it will be? b—I wonder if it will make a difference to our image? c—I wonder when you think you could have it done? d—I wonder what the problem is with our image? e—I wonder if you could tell me if the new logo is ready?)

2. Have students work in pairs to practice saying the indirect questions.

3. (**a**) Divide the class into pairs. Each student reads through the example situations. Make sure all students understand the situations. Then each pair of students adds at least three other situations to the list. Using the language in the model structure, they practice making a request appropriate in each situation. Circulate and monitor content, grammar, and pronunciation. (Answers will vary.)
(**b**) Students swap roles and practice again.

4. (**a**) Give each student time to think of a request that he or she would like to make of someone else in the class. Then tell students to think of a third person whom they will ask to make the request for them. Do one example with the whole class.
(**b**) In pairs, students compare and discuss their responses, then circulate in the class and make their requests.

Self-Check

Communication Challenge

Challenge 8 is on pages 117 and 118 of the student text, and suggestions for its use are on page 117 in this Teacher's Extended Edition.

1. Encourage students to complete this task without looking back at the unit.

2. In this task students work individually and rate their performance on the strategies in this unit. Then they compare and discuss their responses with a partner.

3. You may wish to help students with this task by suggesting some ways in which advertisements try to project an image and sell their product or service. Advertisements may appeal to our sense of family, our desire for security, our desire for value, our desire to be special or different, or our desire to fit in. Ads often appeal because they present a sexy image. Have students bring their advertisements to class to compare and discuss them.

4. Have students work individually to check off the words that they know.

• The grammar summary for this unit is on page 132.

Self-Check

COMMUNICATION CHALLENGE

Group Work Student A: Look at Challenge 8A on page 117. Student B: Look at Challenge 8B on page 118. Student C: Look at Challenge 8C on page 120.

1 Write three new sentences or questions you learned.

....

....

....

2 These are some of the strategies you practiced in this unit. How well can you do these things? Check [√] your answers and then compare with another student.

HOW WELL DID YOU DO?

	Excellent	Good	So-so	Need more practice
• **Selective listening** (listening for the most important words and information)	☐	☐	☐	☐
• **Practicing** (listening or reading and repeating—practicing improves your fluency and makes you a better speaker)	☐	☐	☐	☐
• **Memorizing conversational patterns** (learning phrases to start conversations and keep them going)	☐	☐	☐	☐

3 Out of Class Find examples of advertisements that are being used to develop particular images for the products they are selling. These can be in English or in your own language. Bring them to class and discuss the image the company is trying to project, how they have tried to do this, and how successful they have been.

4 Vocabulary check. Check [√] the words you know.

Adjectives/Adverbs		Nouns		Verbs		
☐ confined	☐ incompetent	☐ answering machine	☐ latter	☐ compare	☐ stop	☐ keep on
☐ corporate	☐ increased		☐ logo	☐ confirm	☐ tolerate	☐ lay off
☐ difficult	☐ indirect	☐ calling services	☐ manufacturer	☐ continue	☐ transfer	☐ look forward to
☐ distinctive	☐ luxury	☐ communications	☐ mobile phone	☐ convey	**Phrasal Verbs**	☐ move in
☐ environmentally-friendly	☐ negative	☐ connotation	☐ morale	☐ convince	☐ call up	☐ plan on
	☐ obtainable	☐ consultant	☐ plan	☐ design	☐ cut down on	☐ put off
☐ faulty	☐ occasionally	☐ corporation	☐ quality	☐ dispatch	☐ get through	☐ put up with
☐ further	☐ valuable	☐ dating service	☐ scenario	☐ forward	☐ get out	☐ stay in
☐ identifying		☐ elegance	☐ slogan	☐ postpone	☐ give up	☐ take up
		☐ expression	☐ solutio	☐ rank	☐ go through with	
		☐ fax	☐ products	☐ recommend		
		☐ image	☐ voice mail			
		☐ intentions				

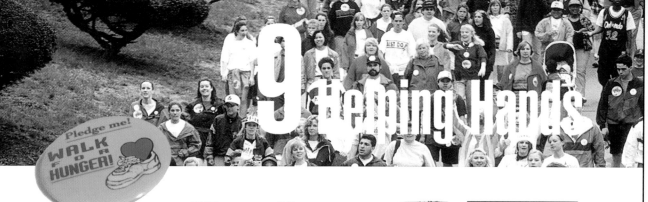

9 Helping Hands

Warm-Up

Unit Goals

In this unit you will:

Ask others to do things

"I'd like you to support Greenpeace."

"I want you to take a few minutes to read this brochure."

Make excuses

"I'm sorry, but I seem to be out of cash right now."

Talk about hypothetical situations in the past

"If it had been me, I'd have changed jobs."

"Well, I think that the first picture has to do with raising money for education."

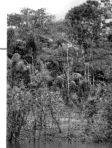
Picture 1

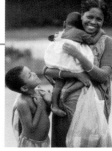
Picture 2

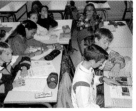
Picture 3

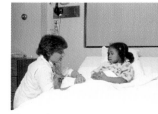
Picture 4

1 **Group Work** These pictures are from organizations that raise money for different causes. Can you think of a cause for each of these pictures?

2 a **Group Work** Discussion. These are excerpts from letters asking for money for charitable causes. Can you match each excerpt with a picture?

.... Just ten dollars will feed a child for . . .

.... is now a major health issue in every country in the . . .

.... We need your help to save the endangered . . .

.... to provide books and materials for those who can't afford them.

b **Pair Work** Take turns making the excerpts into complete sentences.

□ Student text page 67

Warm-Up

Unit Goals. This section presents the language of asking others to do things, making excuses, and talking about hypothetical situations. Have individual students read aloud each of the goals and the examples. Ask students to indicate those that they feel they can do in English.

1. Have students do this task in small groups. They should describe what they see in the picture and, using the sample language as a model, say what cause it suggests to them. Circulate and monitor grammar and pronunciation.
(Suggested answers: 1—the environment; 2—Third World poverty; 3—underprivileged children; 4—critically ill children)

2. **(a)** With the whole class, read through each of the extracts. Then have students work in groups to discuss what words and/or phrases in each fragment give them a clue to the cause that is referred to.
(Answers, top to bottom: Picture 2; Picture 4; Picture 1; Picture 3)
(b) With the whole class, make a complete sentence from one of the fragments. Then have students work in pairs to write a complete sentence for each of the others. Call on students at random to read a statement to the class.
(Answers will vary.)

Task Chain 1: A charitable cause

Learning Strategy. Brainstorming is an important way for students not only to give their own ideas and opinions but also to hear those of other learners. In this way they become familiar with different ways of looking at things and other ways of learning.

Task 1. (a) In this task students read for specific information—that is, key words or phrases that link the text to one of the pictures. Give students enough time to read the text individually and decide which picture matches it.
(Answer: Picture 2)
　(b) With the whole class, discuss ways that students could support a cause such as Oxfam. Make sure they use the sample language as a model. Circulate and check pronunciation and grammar. **Variation.** Allow students to discuss another cause of their choosing.

Task 2. (a) ∩ Play the tape, pausing after each person. Students listen and match one of the pictures with each conversation. **Optional.** Play the tape again and have students write down the key words that helped them decide.
(Answers [left to right]: first picture—Conversation 1; second picture—Conversation 4; third picture—Conversation 3)
　(b) ∩ An important listening skill is understanding how information in spoken language is organized. In this task students work individually and listen for the name of each charity mentioned and the kind of work it does. Play the tape several times if necessary. Elicit answers from around the class.
(Answers: Linda—Educare, which helps impoverished children finish high school; Mike—Everett Foundation, which raises money for AIDS education; Martha—Blue Star Charity Appeal, which does volunteer work in the Third World; Peter—World Youth Fund, which promotes international understanding among the young)
　(c) ∩ Play the tape once more. Have students listen in pairs and then write down the reactions of the people approached for the charities.

(Continued on page 69.)

Task Chain 1 A charitable cause

LEARNING STRATEGY

Brainstorming = thinking of as many new words and ideas as you can.

A Let's have a 24-hour fast to raise money for Oxfam.

B How does that work?

A Well, you get friends and family to sponsor you. They donate a dollar for every hour you can last without food.

Task 1

a Read the following text and match it with a picture from page 67.

On May 8, you may be taking your mother out to lunch to thank her for her years of devotion to your health and happiness. This year, for the cost of that meal, you could give a Mother's Day gift to hundreds of mothers in the developing world. Women who care as much about their children as your mother does about you, but who have to fight hard every day just to find enough food to feed them. But you can help change that with a donation to Oxfam in your mother's name. Oxfam teaches women to read and write, helps them to improve their livestock-raising skills, and offers loans to launch a family business. All this benefits the whole community. This Mother's Day, don't just take your mother out to lunch. Give her a gift she'll really appreciate—the opportunity to help change the lives of mothers around the world. For every donation received by May 3, we will send you a special card to give your mother for Mother's Day on May 8.

b **Group Work** Brainstorm. Think of other ways of supporting causes such as Oxfam.

Task 2

a ∩ Listen. You will hear four people raising money for charitable causes. Match the conversations and the pictures.

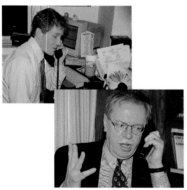

Conversation ...2......

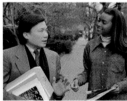

Conversation ...1.....

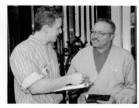

Conversation ......4....

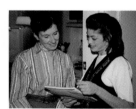

Conversation .3......

b ∩ Listen again. What is the name of each charity? What kind of work does the charity do?

PERSON	NAME OF CHARITY	WORK IT DOES
Linda		
Mike		
Martha		
Peter		

c 🎧 **Pair Work** Listen once more and note the reactions of the people being approached. Complete these statements.

People's Reactions

.... 1 The person approached by Linda reacted by ....

.... 2 The person approached by Mike reacted by ....

.... 3 The person approached by Martha reacted by ....

.... 4 The person approached by Peter reacted by ....

d **Pair Work** Rank the reactions from most to least favorable (1 to 4).

e **Group Work** Discussion. Whose views are most like or least like yours? How would you have reacted in each case?

"Well, I think that . . . got the most
favorable reaction."

"I agree. And . . . got the least
favorable reaction."

Task 3

a Which of the following causes do you think is the most important internationally? Which is most important in your country?

b **Group Work** Can you add to the list? Now fill in the chart by putting a check [√] to rate the importance of each cause.

	IN YOUR COUNTRY			INTERNATIONALLY		
	a little	no	yes	a little	no	yes
World hunger						
Saving the environment						
Research into public health problems						
Helping political prisoners						
....						
....						

c **Group Work** Discuss your choices. Give reasons.

Task 4

a **Group Work** Brainstorm. Make a list of all the things in your school or neighborhood that you could collect money for.

b **Group Work** Now brainstorm ideas for raising money for one of these causes (a fun run, a walkathon, an art exhibition).

c **Group Work** Compare ideas. Which group had the most interesting ones?

Task 5

a Write a letter seeking support for one of the causes from Task 3.

b **Pair Work** Exchange letters and write a response.

Dear Community Member,

Tania Koslowski is one of the most gifted athletes our school has ever seen. She has just been selected for the International Junior Athletics meet in Helsinki. We want you to consider sponsoring Tania to go to Helsinki in July.

We ....
....
....

📖 Student text pages 68–69 (cont.)

(Answers: 1—saying that he didn't have time; 2—slamming down the phone; 3—asking how much to give; 4—offering thirty dollars)

(d) Still in pairs, students decide which of the characters got the best/worst reactions from the people they approached and rank the reactions. Check responses around the class.

(Answers [most to least favorable]: Peter, Martha, Linda, Mike)

(e) Students, in groups, discuss the views expressed on the tape and compare them to their own opinions. Students then speculate on what they would have done in the same situation.

Task 3.   (a) Have each student think about which cause is most important in the world and which cause is most important in their country. Have them compare their responses with those of at least two other students.

(b) In small groups, students try to think of other causes to add to the list and then rate each cause as to its importance.

(c) In the same groups, students discuss their choices.

Task 4.   (a) In small groups, students brainstorm things in their school or neighborhood that they could collect money for.

(b) Go through the examples and make sure that the students understand these fund-raising activities. Then, in small groups, students compare and discuss their ideas for raising money for one or more of the causes in their list.

(c) Combine two groups to compare and discuss ideas. Then, with the whole class, decide which group had the most interesting or original ideas.

Task 5.   (a) Have students do this as an individual writing task. Encourage students to write a rough draft of their letter. Check spelling and grammar. Then have them produce their second/final draft, incorporating your corrections. With the whole class, decide who the letter is being sent to and then complete the request.

(b) In pairs, students exchange and read each other's letter and write a reply, once again using two drafts. Then ask students to read the reply to their original letter and discuss their reaction to it.

Language Focus 1: Object + infinitive

1. **(a)** Give students enough time to read the requests and responses at least twice. Then have them work individually to match them.
(Answers: 1. Oh, dear, I've left my glasses at home. 2. I already did—last week. 3. But Gina and Andre aren't here today. 4. I'm afraid they think it's a waste of money. 5. I'm not sure that we have the time. 6. I thought they only wanted people with talent.)

(b) Make sure the requests and responses are correctly completed before pairs of students begin to practice them. Remind students that this is an opportunity for speaking practice. If possible, they should practice the exchanges by memorizing them rather than reading them.

2. **(a)** Have students work individually to complete the statements.
(Suggested answers: 1—the man to pledge money to a charity; 2—him to go away; 3—the woman to examine her group's brochure; 4—he wanted the man to support the World Youth Fund)

(b) Have students work in pairs to compare their answers. Play the tape again, if necessary.

3. Since this is quite a challenging task, you may want to do one or two examples with the whole class. Point out that to create an appropriate request, students need to look for key words/clues in the excuses. Working in pairs, students write a request for each of the excuses. Make this a collaborative writing task. Each pair produces just one set of requests. Circulate and correct spelling and grammar. Call on several students to read out one of their requests.

4. **(a)** Have students jot down their ideas about each of the requests. In particular, have students consider what communication strategies they would use in each situation. Circulate and provide help as necessary.

(b) Have students work in small groups to decide what the appropriate response would be to each request. Then they practice the situation. Make sure that each student plays both parts.

Language Focus 1 Object + infinitive

1 **a** Match these requests and responses.

Requests
1 I'd like you just to read this promotional brochure.
2 I want you to think about giving to the Freedom from Hunger Campaign.
3 We need everyone to sign the petition on human rights.
4 I want you to talk to your friends about the Environmental Aid Appeal.
5 I'd like you and Alicia to help us raise money for the library fund.
6 They want us to take part in the charity concert.

Responses
.... I'm afraid they think it's a waste of money.
.... Oh, dear, I don't have my glasses with me.
.... I thought they only wanted people with talent.
.... I'm not sure that we have the time.
.... But Gina and Andre aren't here today.
.... I already did—last week.

b **Pair Work** Now practice the requests and responses with a partner.

2 **a** Look at the chart in Task 2b (page 68) and complete these statements following the model at left.

1 Linda wanted ....
2 The person talking to Mike wanted ....
3 Martha asked ....
4 Peter said ....

b **Pair Work** Compare your answers. (You may listen again if necessary.)

3 **Pair Work** Think of requests that might elicit these excuses.

a I'm sorry, the phone is out of order.
b Oh, there's my bus. I've got to run.
c I left my planner at home, but I think I'm busy next Tuesday night.
d I'm not going to school tomorrow either.
e I'd love to, but my wife wouldn't approve.

4 **a** Make notes on what you would have to say to do these things.

1 Ask a stranger to donate to a charity that helps homeless children.
2 Get a friend to help you collect money for your favorite charity.
3 Get the rest of the class to take part in a walk against cancer.

b **Group Work** Now take turns role playing each situation.

"We wanted the teachers to support our school bus campaign."

A I'd like you to call the bank for me.
B I'm sorry, the phone is out of order.

Task Chain 2 — Harry the helper

Task 1

a **Group Work** Imagine that you are one of these people. Make up a story about the picture and tell it to the group.

b Select the most interesting/funniest story and tell it to the class. Which group has the best story?

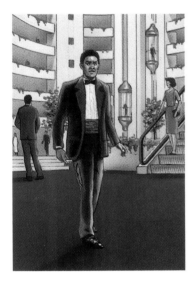
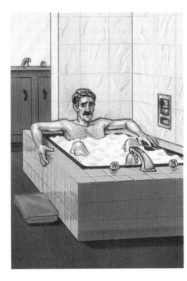
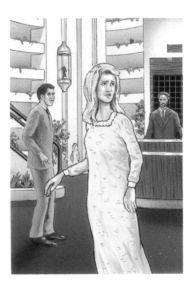

Task 2

a 🎧 Listen to the conversation. Which of the incidents in Task 1 are described?

b 🎧 Listen again and fill in the chart.

"If Harry hadn't helped the VIP, he'd have been . . . "

INCIDENT	WHAT HAPPENED	WHAT HARRY DID
VIP		
groom		
celebrity		

c **Pair Work** Take turns saying what would have happened if Harry hadn't helped.

Task Chain 2: Harry the helper

Task 1. (a) The pictures in this task provide the context and framework for the recounting of an incident. Students may choose to be a secondary character in the story rather than the protagonist.

(b) Allow students to circulate and listen to the stories being told in other groups. Have them vote on the one that they find most interesting, and then ask for a volunteer to retell it to the class.

Task 2. (a) 🎧 Play the tape. Students listen to see if the conversation describes the people shown in the pictures.

(Answers: elderly, wealthy looking gentleman lying in bath, with toe stuck in faucet; man dressed for wedding but with large tear in pants; famous actress in lobby sleepwalking in her nightgown)

(b) 🎧 Play the tape again. Stop the tape after each incident to give students time to make notes. Then they fill in the chart.

(Answers: VIP—got his toe stuck in a faucet; Harry sprayed the toe with a special lubricant. Groom—split his pants; Harry lent the guest his own pants. Celebrity—came into the hotel lobby wearing only a nightgown; Harry realized that she was sleepwalking and took her by the arm and led her back to her room.)

(c) Remind students of the rule for sentences of this type: *had* + past participle in the *if* clause and *would have* + past participle in the main clause. In pairs, students complete the example and then write *if* sentences for the other two. Circulate and correct spelling and grammar. When the sentences are correct, have students practice saying them. Circulate and check pronunciation.

Task 3. (a) Have students work in groups of three. Each student chooses one of the three incidents recounted in Task 2. (You may need to play the tape again.) Make it clear that students are to rewrite what happened in their own words. Have students write a first/rough draft. Circulate and correct spelling and grammar. Then have students write a second/final draft incorporating your corrections.

(b) In the same groups, students combine their three paragraphs into one complete article. This will mean using joining sentences or clauses.

(c) Make sure that the articles have been corrected for spelling and grammar before students swap with another group and read each other's work.

Task 4. (a) Learning tasks are more successful when learners have a specific focus. Guide this task by determining with the class some ways in which people help others—for example, helping in an emergency, saving someone whose life is in danger, helping others by giving money, helping others do something they can't do. Each student tells the group about a person and why he or she should be honored for helping others.

(b) Have each group vote on which of the people described most deserves an award, and what that award should be.

Task 5. Give students time to think about what they will recount. Guide them to think about a specific situation or time in their life. It might be from the present, the recent past, or years before. Then students tell their story to the others in their group, covering each of the three discussion points and using the sample language as a guide.

Task 3

a **GroupWork** Working with two other students, complete the second paragraph of the following newspaper account using one of the incidents from Task 2. (Each student chooses a different incident.)

Special Award to Harry the Helper

SANTA MONICA The United Hoteliers Association held its 40th Annual Awards Dinner at the Santa Monica Prince Hotel yesterday. A highlight of the evening was the presentation of a special award to Harry Marciano, known throughout the industry as "Harry the Helper." After more than 50 years in the hotel business, Harry has finally decided to hang up his tie and tails. The award was given to Harry in recognition of his years of service, and for bringing new standards of service to the industry.

In making the award, Association President Ruth DeVries recounted several of Harry's better-known exploits. For instance, there was the time that

_____
_____
_____
_____
_____
_____
_____
_____

b **GroupWork** Use your paragraphs to produce a complete article.

c **GroupWork** Compare articles with another group.

Task 4

a **GroupWork** Think of someone you know who deserves an award for helping others. Tell the group about this person, giving reasons why he or she should be honored.

b **GroupWork** Vote on the most deserving person and think of an appropriate award for them.

Task 5

GroupWork Think of a time that you have been helped by someone else. Tell the story to the group. Describe (1) the problem you had, (2) the help you received, and (3) what would/wouldn't have happened if you hadn't gotten help.

"I once went to visit a friend in a strange town and he'd gone away for the weekend. I didn't have enough money to stay in a hotel, and I would have been in big trouble if a nice couple hadn't let me stay in their apartment overnight."

Language Focus 2 Past conditional

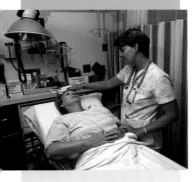

1 **Pair Work** Match the two halves of the statements and practice them.

a If I hadn't become a nurse,
b If I'd become an attorney,
c If I'd stayed in social work,
d If I hadn't gone into teaching,
e If I'd stayed in school,

.... I would have become rich.
.... I wouldn't have ended up in this dead-end job.
.... I wouldn't have gotten to work with young people.
.... I would probably have become a social worker.
.... I would have worked mostly with elderly people.

2 **Group Work** Compare your responses with three other students.

3 **Pair Work** Some of these sentences are incorrect. Correct them and practice them with a partner.

a I would have made a lot of money if I has stayed in advertising.
b If he had become an attorney, George was a wealthy man today.
c If we had left when I said, we wouldn't have the accident.
d I wouldn't have gone into medicine if I'd known how stressful it was.
e You wouldn't have the job if you hadn't been so convincing in the interview.

4 **Pair Work** Respond to each of the following statements following the model at left.

A Sergio won half a million dollars and spent it all in a year.

B If it had been me, I'd have spent it all in six months.

a Peter got fired, and did nothing about it.
b George was in an accident that was caused by the other person, but decided not to sue.
c Tina left her job because she had too far to commute.
d The airline lost Alison's suitcase on her trip to Mexico, and she never got it back.
e When I accepted the job, they only gave me half the salary they had promised.

"I guess the most important decision I ever made was emigrating. If I hadn't moved to Canada, I would never have learned English."

5 a **Pair Work** What are the three most important decisions you have ever made? What would have happened/not happened if you hadn't made that decision? Tell your partner.

b **Group Work** Tell another pair about your partner's situation.

Language Focus 2: Past conditional

1. Have students work in pairs. Give students time to read each of the partial statements and then match them. Circulate and make sure that their answers are correct before students begin to practice them. (Suggested answers: a—If I hadn't become a nurse, I would have worked with elderly people. b—If I'd become an attorney, I would have become rich. c—If I'd stayed in social work, I would probably have become a social worker. d—If I hadn't gone into teaching, I wouldn't have gotten to work with young people. e—If I'd stayed in school, I wouldn't have ended up in this dead-end job.)

2. Have students compare their responses in small groups.

3. Working in pairs, students read each sentence and see if they can spot the mistake. Elicit answers from around the class. Then have partners practice saying the sentences until they can say them from memory. (Answers: a—*had* stayed in advertising. b—*would be* a wealthy man today. c—wouldn't have *had* the accident. d—how stressful it *would be*. e—wouldn't have *gotten* the job.)

4. With the whole class, read through each of the statements. Then, in pairs, students put themselves into the situation and practice saying what they would do, using the structure "If it had been me, I'd have. . . ." (Answers will vary.)

5. (a) All students bring their own knowledge to the learning, and new learning is successful only if it is linked to this prior knowledge and experience. Guide students to think about important decisions they have made in specific areas of their life. They choose three important decisions they have made and consider how things might have been different if they had made another decision.

(b) Combine two pairs and have each student tell the group about his or her partner's decisions.

Self-Check

Communication Challenge

Challenge 9 is on page 118 of the student text, and suggestions for its use are on that page in this Teacher's Extended Edition.

1. Encourage students to complete this task without looking back at the unit.

2. Students need the opportunity to assess their own progress and make judgments about their own learning. In this task students work individually and rate their performance on the strategies of this unit.

3. Remind students that the You Choose tasks are an important opportunity for them to make some decisions of their own about the learning. Have students who choose **B** decide on and write down the questions that they will ask in the interview. Encourage them to ask the questions, as much as possible, from memory, without referring to the written notes.

4. Have students work individually to check off the words that they know.

•   The grammar summary for this unit is on page 132.

Self-Check

Self-Check

COMMUNICATION CHALLENGE
Look at Challenge 9 on page 118.

1 Write three new sentences or questions you learned.

....

....

....

2 The following are some of the strategies you practiced in this unit. How well can you do these things? Check [√] your answers and then compare with another student.

HOW WELL DID YOU DO?

	Excellent	Good	So-so	Need more practice
Personalizing (sharing your own opinions, feelings, and ideas about a subject)	☐	☐	☐	☐
Brainstorming (thinking of as many new words and ideas as you can)	☐	☐	☐	☐
Cooperating (sharing ideas with other students and learning together)	☐	☐	☐	☐

3 **Out of Class** *You choose:* Do **A** or **B**.

A Collect some material from various charitable organizations or groups. Bring these to class and tell the class about them. Say how they raise money and what they do with the money.

B Find somebody who has been helped out of a difficult situation. Make notes and recount the story to the class.

4 Vocabulary check. Check [√] the words you know.

Adjectives/Adverbs		
☐ charitable	☐ health	☐ sleepwalking
☐ developing	☐ helper	☐ terrible
☐ endangered	☐ homeless	☐ underprivileged
☐ favorable	☐ hypothetical	
☐ gifted	☐ promotional	

Nouns		
☐ appeal	☐ charity	☐ human
☐ attorney	☐ devotion	rights
☐ award	☐ excerpt	☐ petition
☐ brochure	☐ famine	☐ recognition
☐ cause	☐ happiness	☐ relief

Verbs		
☐ appreciate	☐ change	☐ promise
☐ approach	☐ commute	☐ raise
☐ approve	☐ donate	☐ react
☐ benefit	☐ help	☐ sponsor
☐ brainstorm	☐ lose	☐ support

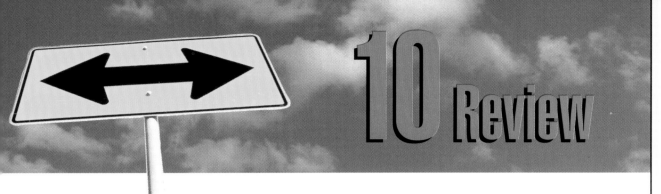

10 Review

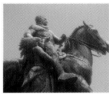
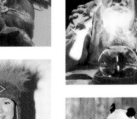
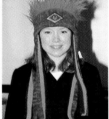
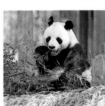

📖 Student text page 75

Task 1

a Underline the words that appeared in Unit 7. Look the others up in your dictionary.

	People	Places	Animals
unusual	☐	☐	☐
exotic	☐	☐	☐
bizarre	☐	☐	☐
extraordinary	☐	☐	☐
ridiculous	☐	☐	☐
frightening	☐	☐	☐
popular	☐	☐	☐
evil	☐	☐	☐
endangered	☐	☐	☐
....	☐	☐	☐
....	☐	☐	☐
....	☐	☐	☐

b Which of these words could you use to describe people, places, or animals? Put a check [√] in the appropriate box.

c **Pair Work** Add three words of your own to the list, and then practice making statements about the pictures.

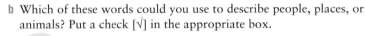

"The man in the cloak is the most frightening person I've ever seen."

Task 2

a Look at these functions. Match them with the pieces of conversation listed below. Write the correct number in the blank.

.... expressing a superlative
.... reporting what someone else said
.... giving a definition
.... making an indirect request
.... making an excuse
.... talking about a hypothetical situation

1 . . . if you could help us to . . .
2 . . . delinquents are kids whose parents . . .
3 . . . I'm sorry but . . .
4 . . . that she had called the day before . . .
5 . . . I wouldn't have been able to buy . . .
6 . . . the most wonderful gift that . . .

b **Pair Work** Think of a situation for each of the phrases. Make up two-line conversations and practice them.

This is the second of three review units. It is designed to consolidate some of the key vocabulary, grammar, and language functions introduced in Units 6–9.

Task 1. (a) Students turn back to Unit 7 and underline the words in the list that appeared there. (Answers: unusual, frightening, endangered)

(b) Each student decides which words could or couldn't be used to describe people, places, and animals. Students mark their answers on the chart. Note that it is often easier to decide what cannot be used, and why not, rather than what can be used and why. (Answers will vary.)

(c) In pairs, students add words to the list. Then students make statements about each of the pictures. Remind them to use the sample language as a guide. **Variation.** Do one example with the whole class first, and then have students make statements about the other pictures.

Task 2. (a) In this task students consider both the form and the meaning of language. Have students do this as an individual writing task, but first review with the whole class each of the functions and make sure that everyone understands them.
(Answers: 1—making an indirect request; 2—giving a definition; 3—making an excuse; 4—reporting what someone else said; 5—talking about a hypothetical situation; 6—expressing a superlative)

(b) In pairs, students think of situations for each of the conversation extracts. Encourage them to be as specific as they can and to consider the context—that is, the situation, what is happening, and who is taking part. Make sure that you allow enough time for this task. Then have students create their own short dialogues. You may decide to allow the discussion to continue for as long as the students are interested and actively involved. Circulate and correct grammar and content before students use the dialogues for speaking practice.

Task 3. (a) ∩ Play the tape once and have students listen for and write down the inventions discussed. Play the tape a second time and have students write down the reasons why the inventions were invented. (Answers: 1—Super-Loop Plug; to make it easier to get the plug out of a bathtub. 2—Post-it® Note; for occasions when something doesn't need to stick permanently. 3—suction hooks; so that items could be attached to walls without scarring them)

(b) In pairs, students make statements about the three inventions. Make sure that they use the sample language.

Task 4. (a) Read each response aloud at least twice. Review with the class how indirect questions are formed. In this task students create their own language from models and examples they have been working with. Give students several minutes to think of an appropriate indirect request for each response—that is, what they will ask and how (the exact words they will use).
(Answers will vary.)

(b) In pairs, students role-play making the requests and responding to them. Make sure that all students play each part. Circulate and check content and pronunciation.

Task 5. (a) This task looks at expressing hypothetical actions. In pairs, students read the letter at least twice. They discuss the blanks and what they would do in each case. Then they complete the letter. Circulate and correct grammar and spelling.

(b) Have students work in groups. Tell students to ask their partners about unlucky things that have happened to them or to someone they know. Students then consider what they would have done in the same situation. They may decide they would have done the same thing that the other person did, or they may have done something different.

Task 3

a ∩ Listen. You will hear people talking about three inventions. In the chart, make a note of the inventions and the reasons why they were invented.

INVENTION	WHY INVENTED
1	
2	
3	

b **Pair Work** Now make statements about each invention using the model at left.

"The . . . was invented/created/devised . . ."

A: I wonder if you'd like to play tennis on Saturday?

B: I'm sorry, but it's my boyfriend's birthday.

Task 4

a Study the following responses to some indirect requests. Think of appropriate requests and write them in the spaces provided.

Indirect Request	*Response*
1	"I'm afraid I can't. I just used the last one myself."
2	"Sure. I'll pick them up after school."
3	"Not at all. Here you are."
4	"I'm sorry, but my parents are visiting this weekend."
5	"I'm sorry, but I need it myself today."

b **Pair Work** Practice the requests and responses.

Task 5

a **Pair Work** Read this letter and take turns saying what you would have done in each situation.

It was the worst vacation ever. We arrived at the airport, and they wouldn't let us board the plane because neither of us had visas for Australia (our travel agent had told us we didn't need them!) So ....

When we finally got there, we discovered that because of a strike, there was no transportation into the city ....

Our problems continued when we got to the hotel. Because our flight had been delayed, the hotel had given away our room, and they said that they were completely booked. So we decided to ....

After everything was figured out, we got to our room, and I discovered that I'd left my briefcase with my computer and all my papers in the taxi. ....

b **Group Work** Ask group members about unfortunate things that have happened to them and say what you would have done in those situations.

11 Speaking Personally

Unit Goals

In this unit you will:

Ask for personal information
"What do you enjoy doing most?"

Express attitudes and opinions
"I think that growing up in a happy, secure environment is more important than growing up in a wealthy environment."

"In five years, the guy at the desk will be retired."

Warm-Up

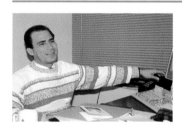
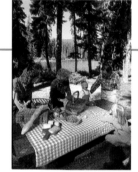
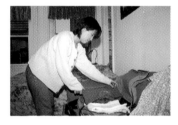
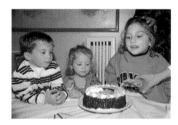

1 **Group Work** Discussion. Look at these people. What are they doing? What do you think they'll be doing . . .

- in a few minutes?   • next year?
- next week?   • in five years?

2 **Group Work** Discussion. What do you think that you will be doing in the time periods listed above?

3 **a** Select three words from this list that best describe you.

ambitious	relaxed	aggressive	tense	easygoing
intense	patient	hard-working	fun-loving	competitive
friendly	lazy	impatient		

b Now compare your evaluations with another student.

c Which of these words do you think describe the people in the pictures?

Speaking Personally   **77**

Student text page 77

Warm-Up

Unit Goals. This section presents the language of asking for personal information and expressing attitudes and opinions. Choose individual students to read aloud each of the goals and the examples. Have students indicate those that they feel they can do in English.

1. It is important for learners to give their opinions and hear those of others and to speculate from their own knowledge and experience. In this task students, in groups, first say what the people in the photographs are doing.
(Answers will vary. Suggested answers: top left—working in an office; top right—having a family picnic; bottom left—packing for a trip; bottom right—celebrating a birthday.)
Then students share their views about what they think the people in the pictures might be doing in the future and why they think so. The objective of the discussion is to share ideas and opinions, not to arrive at consensus.

2. Students speculate on what they will be doing at different points in time, from a few minutes up through five years. Encourage them to think about what they would like to be doing and balance that with what they think is most likely to happen.

3. (a) Read through the list of words with the whole class to make sure that all students understand them. Then each student chooses three adjectives to describe him- or herself. **Variation.** Have each student choose three words to describe another student in the class. Then have students discuss their description with the person that they have described.
(b) In pairs, students compare and discuss their self-descriptions. **Variation.** Students choose three words to describe their partner.
(c) Students consider the pictures and choose words to describe each person.

Speaking Personally   **77**

Task Chain 1: Talking about ourselves

Task 1. (a) Working in pairs, students share their personal views about the qualities they would look for in someone with whom they were going to do these activities. Encourage students to give reasons for their opinions. The objective of the discussion is to share ideas and opinions, not to arrive at consensus.

(b) With the whole class, brainstorm aspects of people's appearance or behavior that students think reveal something about the person. List these on the board. Then have students work in pairs to develop their questions, using the sample language as a model.

Task 2. (a) Working individually, students answer each of the questions, using the sample language as a guide. **Variation.** Have students do this as an individual writing task. Circulate and correct grammar and spelling.

(b) Have students work in pairs to compare their responses. Circulate and check grammar and pronunciation.

(c) Working individually, students write two additional questions. Check to see that spelling and grammar are correct before students, in pairs, ask and answer the questions.

Task 3. (a) 🎧 Play the tape. Pause after each interview to allow students to take notes. Then play all three interviews again so that students can verify their responses.
(Answers: Mark—1. Play the banjo. 2. To be as good a player as Doc Boggs. 3. Learning how to write computer programs. 4. How Doc Boggs plays the banjo. 5. Being able to buy a house in the mountains. 6. Traveling to India. Vanessa—1. Writing stories. 2. To be happy and successful. 3. Getting her present job. 4. Her mother. 5. Her job. 6. Winning a design competition. Sylvia—1. Lying on the beach. 2. To do more enjoyable things. 3. Learning to speak modern Greek. 4. One of her old professors. 5. Moving to Toronto. 6. Meeting Marilyn Horne.)

(b) Students consider which of the people interviewed is most/least like them. Ask for responses from around the class.

Task Chain 1 Talking about ourselves

"Well, I'd ask what clothes they like to wear when they're relaxing, because that says a lot about someone's personality—you know, if they're laid back or not."

"What do I like doing more than anything else? Just hanging out with my friends, I guess."

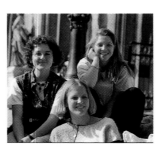

Task 1

a **Pair Work** Discussion. What qualities would you look for in someone you were going to . . .

- go on a vacation with?
- share an apartment with?
- complete a work/school project with?
- buy a car from?

b **Pair Work** What questions would you ask to identify these qualities?

Task 2

a Answer the following questions.

1 What do you enjoy doing more than anything else?
2 What is your greatest ambition in life?
3 What is your greatest achievement so far?
4 Who do you admire most in the world, and why?
5 What is the best thing that has ever happened to you?
6 What is the most exciting thing that has ever happened to you?

b **Pair Work** Compare your responses with another student's responses.

c Add two questions to the list in Task 2a and survey another student.

Task 3

a 🎧 Listen to the tape and make a note of the answers these people give to the questions.

QUESTION	MARK	VANESSA	SYLVIA
1			
2			
3			
4			
5			
6			

b Which person is most like you? Which person is least like you?

c **Group Work** Discussion. Work with three or four other students and complete this survey.

	MARK			VANESSA			SYLVIA		
Which of these people would you . . .	YES	MAYBE	NO	YES	MAYBE	NO	YES	MAYBE	NO
go on a vacation with?									
share an apartment with?									
complete a work/school project with?									
buy a car from?									

LEARNING STRATEGY

Role playing =
pretending to be
someone else and using
the right language for
the situation you are in.

d **Group Work** Think of questions you would like to ask each person. Role play the questions and answers.

Task 4

a **Pair Work** The following resume was written by Mark, Vanessa, or Sylvia. Write his/her name in the blank space.

.... Byrne

2618 Calcaterra Drive
Santee, California 92071

EDUCATION   1989— High School Diploma,
              Mosswood High School

              1991— Diploma in graphic design,
              San Jose Vocational College

EXPERIENCE   1992–1993 Trainee designer,
              Graphart Design, San Francisco

              1993–1994 Designer and editor,
              Latin America Editores, Mexico City

              1994 to present Graphic designer,
              In Press, San Jose

INTERESTS   Music of all kinds, modern literature,
              painting, languages, and travel.

b **Group Work** Write your own resume but don't put your name on it. Give it to the teacher and take someone else's resume. Can you guess who wrote the resume you have?

(c) Make sure that the groups discuss each of the questions and complete the survey. Manage the discussion so that those students who usually talk less can give their opinions.

(d) The groups work to come up with at least three questions to ask each of the interviewees. Have students practice asking and answering these in a role play.

Learning Strategy.   Role playing gives students the opportunity to practice different styles of language and to change their language to suit a range of different language situations or contexts.

Task 4.   (a) Give students time to read the resume at least twice. Then, in pairs, they discuss who they think it was written by.
(Answer: Vanessa)

(b) Begin this as an individual writing task. Using Vanessa's resume as a model, each student writes his or her own. Circulate and check grammar and spelling. Gather the completed resumes (minus names) and redistribute them so that each student has someone else's and then must try to guess who wrote it.

Language Focus 1: *Wh-* questions + gerund/infinitive

1. Remind students that this is a speaking practice task. Developing short-term memory is an important part of learning a new language. Have students read through all the questions to remember them. Then, in pairs, they practice asking and answering the questions from memory.

2. This task involves students in actively thinking about how English works. Rather than simply being given a rule, students are encouraged to use examples and models to recognize language patterns and work out grammar/language rules for themselves.
(Answers: a—to do; b—doing; c—doing; d—doing; e—to do)

Do you know the rule?   (Answers will vary.)

3. (a) Working individually, students correct the mistakes. Go through the answers with the whole class.
(Answers: 1—correct; 2—enjoy doing; 3—correct; 4—hope to go; 5—correct; 6—deny being)
(b) With a partner, students practice asking and answering each of the questions. Circulate and check grammar and pronunciation.

4. (a) In pairs, students write their own survey questions, using the suggestions. Have them do a rough draft of their survey first. Correct grammar and spelling, and then have students write a final draft incorporating your corrections.
(b) Combine pairs and have students survey one another. Remind students that surveys like this are a good way to find out more about their classmates and that they also create a friendly and supportive learning environment. In addition, surveys are speaking practice tasks and give opportunities for learners to be involved in meaningful communication.
(c) An important language skill is being able to report what happened. Have students talk in groups about what they found out about the pair of students that they interviewed, using the sample language as a model.

Language Focus 1 *Wh-* questions + gerund/infinitive

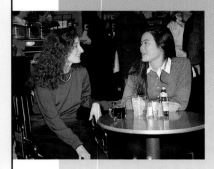

1 **Pair Work** Take turns asking and answering these questions.

a What did you consider doing after graduation?
b Where do you intend to go for your next vacation?
c What did you want to be when you grew up?
d When do you enjoy playing sports?
e Where do you hope to live eventually?
f What kind of music do you dislike listening to most?
g When do you expect to stop taking English classes?
h Where would you suggest going this weekend?
i What chores would you avoid doing if you had the choice?

2 Use the correct form of 'do' (*doing* or *to do*) to complete these statements.

a What did you expect her .... about her job?
b When did he avoid .... the personality survey?
c What did you deny .... yesterday?
d Why did you suggest .... more studying this weekend?
e How did he expect you .... your homework?

3 a Some of these questions are incorrect. Correct them.

1 What do you suggest to do tonight?
2 What do you enjoy to do most on your vacation?
3 Who would you consider bringing to the party?
4 When do you hope going out?
5 What is something you dislike doing by yourself?
6 How could you deny to be at the party when everyone saw you?

b **Pair Work** Now practice them by asking and responding to the questions with another student.

4 a **Pair Work** Make up your own survey using these words plus a gerund (verb + *ing*) or infinitive (*to* + verb).

Who	do/did you	avoid	.... ?
What	do/did you	expect	.... ?
Where	do/did you	hope	.... ?
When	do/did you	consider	.... ?
Why	do/did you	intend	.... ?
How	do/did you	dislike	.... ?
		enjoy	.... ?
		want	.... ?

b **Group Work** Survey another pair.

c **Group Work** Now report the results to a third pair.

Do you know the rule?

Study the examples in this Language Focus and fill in the chart.
Always followed by gerund (-ing)
Example:
finish _____
_____
_____

Always followed by infinitive (to + verb)
Example:
appear _____
_____
_____
_____

"Rama expects to go to the tennis tournament this weekend."

Task Chain 2 Why are we made that way?

Task 1

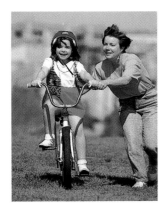

a Pair Work A number of famous people were questioned about their childhood and the things that influenced them. Here are their responses. Can you think of the questions?

1 .... ? "A bike, when I was six years old."
2 .... ? "My mother, because she taught me to get the most out of every day."
3 .... ? "I guess being part of a large happy family."
4 .... ? "Being the only girl in a house full of boys."
5 .... ? "My grandparents' farm."
6 .... ? "Being in a bad car accident when I was around fourteen."

b Pair Work Take turns asking your partner some of the questions. Give answers that are true for you.

Task 2

a 🎧 Listen. You will hear three short conversations. What do/did these people want to do? What things influenced them? Fill in the chart.

NAME	WANTED TO DO/ INFLUENCES	AGE	CURRENT OCCUPATION
Ellie			
Charles			
Mary			

b 🎧 Listen again. Can you guess how old each speaker is? What do you think each person does (or, if it is a child, is likely to do)? Write your answers in the chart.

c Group Work Compare your results, and give reasons.

Task 3

a Skim the text on page 82 and decide which of the following it is. Check [√] one.
☐ a review of a TV program
☐ a magazine article
☐ an excerpt from a book

b Group Work Discussion. Discuss your choice with several other students. What helped you to decide?

Task Chain 2: Why are we made that way?

Task 1. **(a)** Read through each of the answers with the whole class, and offer a question for the first answer. Then, in pairs, students write questions for each of the others. Circulate and correct grammar. Elicit responses from around the class.
(Answers will vary.)

(b) Students choose some of the questions to ask and then take turns asking them. Each student should give answers that are true for him or her.

Task 2. **(a)** 🎧 Play the tape. Working individually, students listen and take notes. Pause the tape after each person to allow students to complete the first column of the table.
(Answers: Ellie—wants to become a genetic engineer because of television program and advice of teacher; Charles—had wanted to become a veterinarian because he loved pets; Mary—had wanted to join the circus because her grandparents had taken her there)

(b) 🎧 All listening involves some personal interpretation of what we hear. But this aspect of listening is often neglected in language teaching. In this task students make judgments about the age of the speaker from the voice quality and from what the speaker says. They also speculate on what course of action each person follows or is likely to follow.
(Answers will vary.)

(c) In groups, students compare and discuss their responses. Circulate and make sure that they give reasons for their choices.

Task 3. **(a)** Have students read the text and then decide where it would be from.
(Answer: a magazine article)

(b) Have students work in small groups to discuss how they made their decision.

(c) Explain to the class that we often use examples from our own or other people's personal experience to support our opinion. In small groups, students discuss what evidence in the text supports the main point, and whether they agree or disagree with it. Then, from their own experience, they provide extra evidence for or against the point.

Task 4. (a) Remind students of the importance of linking the learning to their own lives and opinions. Guide them to think about specific situations or times in their life; then ask them to fill in the chart.

(b) In groups of at least three, students compare and discuss their responses, using the sample language as a model.

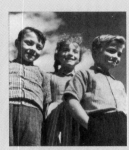

Have you ever thought about what determines the way we are as adults? Remember the documentary series Seven Up? It started following the lives of a group of children in 1963. We first meet them as wide-eyed seven-year-olds and then catch up with them at seven-year intervals: giggling 14-year-olds, earnest 21-year-olds, then mature young adults.

Some of the stories are inspiring, others tragic, but what is striking in almost all the cases is the way in which the children's early hopes and dreams are reflected in their adult lives. For exmple, at seven, Tony is a lively child who says he wants to become a jockey or a taxi driver. When he grows up, he goes on to do both. How about Nicki, who says, "I'd like to find out all about the moon" and goes on to become a rocket scientist. As a child, soft-spoken Bruce says he wants to help "poor children" and ends up teaching in India.

But if the lives of all the children had been this predictable the program would be far less interesting than it actually was. It was the children whose childhood did not prepare them for what was to come that made the documentary so fascinating. Where did their ideas come from about what they wanted to do when they grew up? Are childen influenced by what their parents do, by what they see on television, or by what their teachers say? How great is the impact of a single inspirational event? Many film directors, including Stephen Spielberg, say that an early visit to the local cinema was the turning point in their lives.

Dr. Margaret McAllister, an educational psychologist, confirms that the major influences tend to be parents, friends, and the wider society. "When children first become aware of work, their early choices are unrealistic," says McAllister, "but as they get older, they start to make more realistic choices. Children turn to key role models for inspiration. If we look at imaginative play, it's very common that children play as moms and dads, then once they're at school, teaching becomes a popular choice—they've identified with the teacher, someone who is powerful, in control, and kind."

c **GroupWork** Discussion. What is the main point of the text? What evidence is provided to support that point? Do you agree or disagree? From your own experience, can you think of any evidence for or against the point?

"My grandmother was one of the most influential people in my life because she taught me to get the most out of every single day. The place where we took family vacations was important because it was there that I finally learned to be independent. And graduating from college was important because it enabled me to have the career I wanted."

Task 4

a What have been the three most influential people, places, and events in your life so far? Write in the space provided.

PEOPLE	PLACES	EVENTS
my grandmother	where we took family vacations	graduating from college

b **GroupWork** Now talk about why these people, places, and events were so important.

Language Focus 2 Comparative/superlative + gerund/infinitive

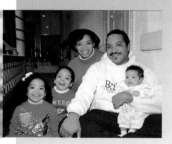

1 **Pair Work** Match these questions and answers and practice them.

Questions
a What did you enjoy most about your early life?
b Why do you say that your teen-age years were boring?
c What was the most important influence on you as a child?
d Why do you say that you fell into this career almost by accident?
e Why do you say you had a more fortunate upbringing than your friends?

Answers
.... Well, it was better to have grown up on a farm, like I did, than in a city apartment, like most of them.
.... There were fewer interesting things to do ten years ago than there are today.
.... Well, for most of my life I'd wanted to be an actor more desperately than a director.
.... The best thing was thinking about what it would be like being an adult.
.... I think being raised by the most artistic and creative parents in the world was the most significant thing.

2 a Complete the following statements using comparatives (*more*) and superlatives (*the most*).

1 Spending a week on a cruise ship in the South Pacific would be .... (comparative).
Spending a week .... would be .... (superlative).
2 To grow up in a .... family would be .... (comparative).
To grow up in a .... family would be .... (superlative).
3 Being a child in .... was .... (comparative).
Being a child in .... was .... (superlative).
4 Living in .... would be .... (comparative).
Living in .... would be .... (superlative).

b **Pair Work** Now practice the statements with a partner.

3 a **Pair Work** Use the structures you've practiced in this Language Focus to make statements about the following topics.

- growing up
- being a child
- being an adult
- living in a large city
- learning another language

b **Pair Work** Take turns having a conversation using as many of these sentences as you can.

- Seeing a good movie would be better than seeing a second-rate concert.
- Seeing the new movie at the Odeon would be the best thing that could happen this weekend.

"Well, I think that growing up in a happy, secure family is the most important thing."

"Well, the best thing about being a child was the fact that it didn't last long! I didn't really like being a kid."

Language Focus 2: Comparative/superlative + gerund/infinitive

1. Have students work in pairs to match the questions and answers. Then have the pairs of students take turns asking and answering the questions. (Answers: a—thinking about being an adult; b—fewer interesting things to do; c—artistic and creative parents; d—had wanted to be an actor; e—better to have grown up on a farm)

2. (a) Go through the first comparison with the whole class and give students time to think about what comparison they will make in each sentence. Then, working individually, students complete each sentence. Circulate and check their responses.
(Answers will vary. Make sure that students use correct comparative and superlative forms and that their sentences are plausible.)
(b) In pairs, students practice their statements, from memory if possible.

3. (a) Have students work in pairs to make statements about the provided topics. Monitor their language structures.
(b) Tell the pairs of students to form a conversation by using the sentences they have created.

Self-Check

Communication Challenge

Challenge 11 is on pages 119 and 121 of the student text, and suggestions for its use are on page 119 in this Teacher's Extended Edition.

1. Encourage students to complete this task without looking back at the unit.

2. (a) In pairs, students discuss their ideas about situations in which they might ask for personal information, and contexts in which they might express their attitude about a situation or an event. Remind students of the importance of linking the learning to their own lives and opinions. Guide them to think about specific situations in their life.

(b) In groups of at least three, students brainstorm ideas about situations in English-speaking countries in which they would have to use this language. Encourage students to think about similar situations they have been in. Circulate and make sure that the suggestions are as specific as possible.

3. Students should make written notes of the questions (see page 78) to help them as they are asking the survey questions. In the interview they should, as much as possible, ask their questions from memory, without referring to the written notes.

4. Have students work individually to check off the words that they know.

- The grammar summary for this unit is on page 133.

Self-Check

COMMUNICATION CHALLENGE

Pair Work Student A: Look at Challenge 11A on page 119. Student B: Look at Challenge 11B on page 120.

1 Write three new sentences or questions you learned.

....
....
....

2 a Review the language skills in this unit. In what situations might you use this language?

WHEN WOULD YOU USE THIS LANGUAGE?

	Situations
Ask for personal information	
Express attitudes and opinions	

b **Group Work** Brainstorm ways to practice this language out of class. Imagine you are visiting an English-speaking country. Where/When might you need this language?

3 **Out of Class** Interview a group of friends or family members using the questions in Task Chain 1, Task 2. Bring the results of your interviews to the classroom and share them with the other students.

Question	Answer
1.	
2	

4 Vocabulary check. Check [√] the words you know.

Adjectives/Adverbs

- aggressive
- ambitious
- competitive
- earnest
- easygoing
- friendly
- fun-loving
- hard-working
- impatient
- inspiring
- intense
- laid back
- lazy
- patient
- personally
- relaxed
- retired
- tense

Nouns

- achievement
- ambition
- anything
- career
- childhood
- choice
- graduation
- influence
- ourselves
- resume
- role model
- scientist
- vacation

Verbs

- admire
- avoid
- complete
- consider
- deny
- dislike
- expect
- express
- hang out
- hope
- intend
- refuse
- role play
- share
- suggest
- want

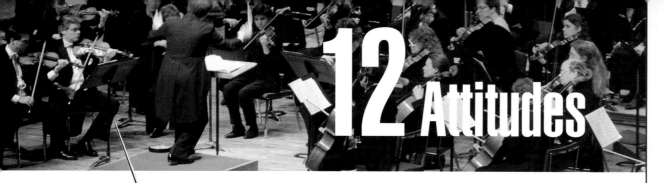

12 Attitudes

Warm-Up

Unit Goals

In this unit you will:

Speculate about future actions
"When my kids are grown they will have done all the things I only dreamed of."

Check and confirm facts and opinions
"You weren't really late for the interview, were you?"

"By this time next week I will have been to my last class of the semester."

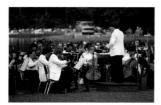
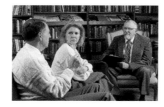
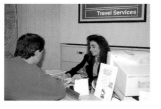
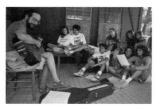

1 a Look up these terms in your dictionary and then write definitions for them in your own words.

Leader: ....
Follower: ....
Advisor: ....

b **GroupWork** Discussion. Look at the pictures and find people who are leaders, followers, and advisors.

2 a Write one thing you plan to have achieved by . . .

- this time tomorrow. ....
- this time next week. ....
- this time next year. ....
- ten years from now. ....

b **GroupWork** Discussion. Share your responses with three or four other students. Who has the most interesting/unusual goals?

📖 Student text page 85

Warm-Up

Unit Goals. This section presents the language of speculating about future actions and checking and confirming facts and opinions. Choose individual students to read aloud each of the goals and the examples. Have students indicate those they feel that they can do in English.

1. (**a**) Elicit answers from individuals around the class.

(**b**) In this task students have the chance to transfer their understanding of dictionary meanings to real-life situations. In small groups, they discuss whether the people depicted in the pictures are leaders, followers, or advisors. Make sure that they give reasons for their choices.

2. (**a**) Give students time to read the statements and decide what they want to have accomplished in the given time frames before writing their answers.

(**b**) Have students work in small groups to discuss their goals. First, give students time to quietly read the work of the others in the group. Then they compare and discuss their answers and, as a group, decide on the most interesting and/or unusual goals.

Task Chain 1: Half full or half empty?

Task 1. (a) Read the expressions to the class at least twice. Give students time to discuss what they understand by these words. Check interpretations with the whole class. Then, after the meanings are clear to everyone, have students decide which expressions describe an optimistic view and which describe a pessimistic view.
(Answers: Optimist—upbeat, up-and-coming; Pessimist—down in the dumps, down side)

(b) Have students do this as an individual reading/writing task. Check answers with the whole class.
(Answers: 1—up-and-coming; 2—down side; 3—down in the dumps; 4—upbeat)

Task 2. (a) Read the statement to the class. Give students time to read through each of the opinions at least twice. Answer any queries. Then have students work in pairs to mark the statements as optimistic or pessimistic. **Optional.** Have individual students say whether they agree or disagree with the statement.
(Answers: Picture 1—O; Picture 2—P; Picture 3—O; Picture 4—P)

Task Chain 1 Half full or half empty?

Task 1

a An optimist is someone who believes that things will turn out well. A pessimist believes that the worst will happen. Which of these expressions would be used by an optimist? Which would you expect to be used by a pessimist? Check [√] your answers.

	Optimist	*Pessimist*
▪ upbeat	☐	☐
▪ down in the dumps	☐	☐
▪ up-and-coming	☐	☐
▪ down side	☐	☐

b Use the expressions to complete these statements.

1 They say that she's an .... actress.
2 The .... of the job are the long hours I have to work.
3 She is .... about losing her job.
4 I'm feeling really .... about prospects for the new year.

Task 2

a These people were asked to react to the statement "In the future, things will not be as good as they are today." Write **O** if the person is *optimistic* and **P** if the person is *pessimistic*.

Picture 1

.... I disagree totally. The people I know look at conditions today with hope. They see a light. I think we're at a point where things are beginning to turn around. I feel upbeat. It's slowly getting better, and our children will be able to have a much better life than we have.

Picture 2

.... I agree. We see what is happening now, and we don't believe anything is going to get better—the economy, the environment—probably because of history. Things didn't seem to get better before, and most people don't think they're going to get better now.

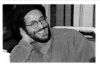
Picture 3

.... We worry about everything in the world, but I think we're still optimistic. We worry about the worst times, but we always have the feeling that we'll be able to do better in the future. If things are bad now, we'll always recover. That's the feeling I have, anyway.

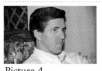
Picture 4

.... Do I see a negative attitude among people today? Yes, I do. It's because of a lack of leadership. People look to their leaders for direction, and they're not getting any. The politicians are not focused.

Source: Adapted from *USA Today*.

b 🎧 Listen to the tape and decide whether the speakers are optimistic or pessimistic. Write (O) or (P) in the chart.

PERSON	OPTIMIST (O)	PESSIMIST (P)	PICTURE NUMBER	KEYWORD(S)
Nicole				
Martin				
Rose				
Edgar				

c 🎧 Listen to the tape again and decide which of the people from Task 2 are talking. Write the picture number in the chart.

d 🎧 Listen once more. Which words gave you clues to the speakers' identities? Write the keywords in the chart.

Task 3

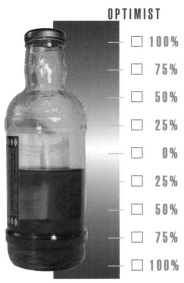

OPTIMIST

☐ 100%
☐ 75%
☐ 50%
☐ 25%
☐ 0%
☐ 25%
☐ 50%
☐ 75%
☐ 100%

PESSIMIST

"Hiroko agrees with the statement. She thinks that there will be fewer job opportunities for young people."

a How optimistic or pessimistic do you think you are? Put a check [√] mark in the appropriate box at left.

b Circle your answers to these questions.

1 What would you say? The bottle is . . .
half full.   half empty.

2 You are taking a trip. Do you assume that the flight will . . .
leave on time?   be delayed?

3 This time next year, do you think that you will be . . .
better off?   worse off?

4 Compared to you, do you think that your children will be . . .
better off?   worse off?

5 You lose your bag. Do you think that the person who finds it will . . .
return it to you?   keep it?

c Based on your answers, are you an optimist or a pessimist?

d **Group Work** Class discussion. Is the class basically optimistic or pessimistic?

Task 4

a **Group Work** Interview three other students. Ask them to agree or disagree with the statement: "In the future, things will not be as good as they are today." Make sure they give you a reason for their opinion. Decide whether they are optimists or pessimists.

b **Group Work** Discuss your findings as a class.

Attitudes **87**

📖 **Student text page 87**

(b) 🎧 Play the tape. Pause the tape after each speaker and allow students to take notes on whether the speaker is optimistic or pessimistic. Play the tape again to let students verify their answers.
(Answers: Nicole—O; Martin—P; Rose—P; Edgar—O)

(c) 🎧 Students listen again to the tape and decide which of the people from Task 2a are talking.
(Answers: Nicole—Picture 1; Martin—Picture 4; Rose—Picture 2; Edgar—Picture 3)

(d) 🎧 Play the tape once more. Students listen for the keywords that told them who each speaker is.
(Suggested answers: Nicole—children, kids; Martin—politicians; Rose—economy, employment, environment; Edgar—future, better)

Task 3. (a) Suggest that students think of one or two recent events in their life and remember how they responded to them. Were they optimistic or pessimistic about what would happen? You may choose to tell them about an incident from your life to show how these attitudes work. Then have students fill in the chart to show how optimistic/pessimistic they are.

(b) Working individually, students complete the quiz.

(c) Elicit responses from around the class about students' self-perception on this issue.

(d) In a whole-class discussion, students compare and discuss their responses. Generalizing from specifics is an important learning skill, and in this task students have the chance to practice it. Elicit the response of each student, and ask students as a whole to figure out whether the class seems more optimistic or more pessimistic, in general.

Task 4. (a) This is a speaking practice task. Before the interviews, give students time to think about how they will answer the question. Then put the class into groups of three, and have students interview each other. During the interview, have the questioners record the responses. This can be done in note form rather than in complete sentences.

(b) Have students report their findings in a whole-class discussion.

Attitudes **87**

Language Focus 1: Future perfect

Learning Strategy.   Explain that practicing is necessary for successful language learning. Students need to practice all four language skills—listening, reading, speaking, and writing.

1. (a) Students work in pairs, with one student reading the first part of the sentence and the other student supplying the end. Make sure that students switch roles so that each member of the pair gets practice in supplying answers.

(b) From their partner's replies, students determine whether the partner is an optimist or a pessimist.

2. (a) Read the sentence beginnings with the whole class. Then have students do the task in two stages. Give them time to think about a prediction for each of the sentences and make notes on it. Then they write their prediction in full. Circulate and correct spelling and grammar. Have students rewrite their predictions, incorporating any corrections you have made.

(b) In pairs, students read each other's statements and then practice saying them. Give students time to practice each one till they can say it from memory.

(c) Combine pairs into groups of four so that each student can relate to the others the predictions of his or her partner.

3. (a) Have students write out their questions before the interview. Give them time to memorize their questions so that they can avoid having to look back at their notes.

(b) Have students take their partner's responses and rephrase them as new statements. Circulate and monitor students' sentences, providing assistance as necessary.

Language Focus 1 Future perfect

Language Focus 1 Future perfect

LEARNING STRATEGY

Practicing = listening or reading and repeating. Practicing improves your fluency and makes you a better speaker.

"Anne says that by the turn of the century, the world population will have increased to ten billion."

"How much television do you watch a day?"

"By the end of the week you'll have watched 28 hours of television."

1 a Pair Work Practice. Take turns saying the first part of each statement. Your partner will complete it using one of the choices given.

  1 By the time the kids get to be my age, the economy will have .... improved. .... deteriorated.

  2 By the end of this year, the world population will have .... doubled. .... stabilized.

  3 This time next year, they .... will .... won't have discovered a cure for cancer.

  4 Ten years from now, we'll all have been made .... unemployed .... wealthy because of technology.

  5 In the next few years, unemployment will have .... risen. .... fallen.

b From his/her answers, is your partner an optimist or a pessimist?

2 a Make some predictions.

  1 This time next week, ...

  2 By the end of this year, ...

  3 This time next year, ...

  4 By the turn of the century, ...

  5 One hundred years from now, ...

b Pair Work Practice the statements with a partner.

c Group Work Tell another pair about your partner's predictions.

3 a Pair Work Interview your partner.

  • time spent watching television per day? ....
  • number of movies seen per month? ....
  • time spent studying or reading per week? ....
  • time spent traveling to work/school per week? ....
  • money spent on food and drink per week? ....
  • time spent talking on telephone per week? ....

b Now make statements about your partner.

Task Chain 2 A born leader

Task 1

a GroupWork Brainstorm. How many qualities can you think of that are associated with *leadership*? Add them to the diagram.

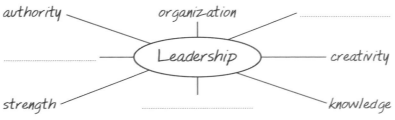

authority — organization

Leadership — creativity

strength — knowledge

b Now use the diagram to make as many statements about leaders as you can.

Example: Leaders are people who . . .

c PairWork What kinds of leadership qualities are desirable in the following types of leaders? List them below.

1 the leader of an athletic organization ....
2 a religious or spiritual leader ....
3 a government leader ....
4 the head of a family ....
5 the head of a corporation ....

Task 2

These advertisement excerpts are from corporations and groups who want to hire people for the following leadership positions. Match the number of the ad to the position.

Positions

.... Coordinator of a new center to help immigrants in an inner city neighborhood

.... Chief conductor of a symphony orchestra

.... High school principal's assistant

.... Someone to take a group of young people on an outdoor adventure vacation in Canada

WE ARE LOOKING for a dynamic person with the right qualifications for this challenging new position. The successful applicant will be a leader who is sensitive to people from many different cultures, who can work with people of all ages, and who is totally committed to equal opportunity for all peoples.

We are looking for a strong but caring leader to take our group in new directions. In addition to creative and artistic skills, you will need to be able to turn a very talented but diverse group of people into a team. You must also be prepared to travel.

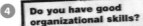
WANTED Caring individual, with leadership potential who is comfortable in the great outdoors. Must like travelling and working with young people. May involve long hours and limited budget.

Do you have good organizational skills? Do you have experience in an educational environment? Do you like working with young people? If so, then you may be the person we are looking for.

Task Chain 2: A born leader

Task 1. (a) Write the word *Leadership* on the board. Have students work in groups to brainstorm qualities they think of when they hear or read this word. Record these on the board. Do not list duplications.

(b) Using the qualities shown in the diagram, students create statements about leadership. This can be a written task, or you could ask for oral answers from volunteers around the room.

(c) With the whole class, read through the list of leaders and do one as an example. Then, in pairs, students discuss the kinds of qualities they think are important for each type of leader in the list and write them in the blanks.

Task 2. This is a scanning task in which students read for specific information. Have them read and mark any words or phrases in the advertisement that they link with any of the positions. Explain that some of the qualities are needed in more than one of the positions. Discuss the answers with the whole class. (Answers: Coordinator—1; Conductor—2; Principal's Assistant—4; Youth Group Leader—3)

Task 3.

(a) 🎧 Play the tape. This is a selective listening task. Students listen only for information that will help them answer the questions. Play the tape more than once if necessary, and allow students to take notes.
(Answer: two people who are interviewing candidates for a position)

(b) 🎧 It is very important for language learners to develop the ability to listen for the main points so that they can summarize what has been said. In this task each student listens to the conversation for positive and negative evaluations of the people talked about. They then summarize what they have heard under the key points listed. Circulate and provide assistance if necessary.
(Answers: Angela—plus; plus; minus; plus; plus. Marty—minus; minus; plus; minus; plus.)

(c) In this task students work in pairs to discuss their personal opinions about the best person for the leadership position and give reasons for their choice.

Task 4.

Remind students that the You Choose tasks are an important opportunity for them to make some decisions of their own about the learning. Read through both tasks with the whole class. Then give students time to consider and choose.

A. Give students time to think of their behavior in each of the situations listed and mark it on the list. Then, in groups, students compare and discuss their lists, using the structure of the sample language. Circulate and monitor content and pronunciation.

B. Students, working in groups, brainstorm names of world, national, or local leaders. They could be political or social leaders, current leaders, or leaders from the past. Each student chooses any of the people from this list and then adds others of his or her own. Students compare and discuss their lists and then negotiate to reduce their combined lists to a new single list.

Task 3

a 🎧 Listen to the conversation. Who is speaking? Who are they discussing?

b 🎧 Listen again and note what is said about each person. Write a (+) for a positive evaluation, and a (−) for a negative evaluation.

	Angela	*Marty*
As a team member, not leader	....	....
Self-motivation	....	....
Ability to delegate	....	....
Attitude toward criticism	....	....
Attitude toward people from other cultures	....	....

c **Pair Work** Discussion. Who do you think is the best person for the leadership position?

Task 4

You choose: Do **A** or **B**

"Well, I'm rarely leader at home, because I'm always being told what to do by the rest of my family."

A People play different roles in different situations. Think of the different roles you play in these situations, and fill in the chart with the appropriate number (1 = often; 2 = sometimes; 3 = seldom; 4 = never).

	AT HOME	AT WORK	AT SCHOOL	WITH FRIENDS
leader				
follower				
planner				
adviser				

Group Work Compare responses and talk about them.

B Make a list of good leaders you have known. What makes each person a good leader?

Group Work Compare lists, then make a single list of essential leadership qualities.

Language Focus 2 Tag questions

Student text page 91

Language Focus 2: Tag questions

Student text page 91

Do you know the rule?

Underline the correct choice.

When the speaker expects a positive answer, he/she uses **a positive tag/a negative tag**.

When the speaker expects a negative answer, he/she uses **a positive tag/a negative tag**.

A You have to travel a lot in your job, don't you?

B Yes, I do.

or

B Well, no, I don't, as a matter of fact.

A You weren't particularly late for the interview, were you?

B Yes, I was, actually. I got off at the wrong subway stop and had to walk further than I'd anticipated.

---

1 a Are these speakers expecting a *yes* or *no* answer? Circle your choice.

1 "You have to travel a lot in your job, don't you?"   Yes   No

2 "She hasn't demonstrated many leadership qualities, has she?"   Yes   No

3 "She has never extended herself at work, has she?"   Yes   No

4 "He should have given more detailed answers, shouldn't he?"   Yes   No

5 "You were in school with my sister, weren't you?"   Yes   No

6 "I guess we've applied for the same position, haven't we?"   Yes   No

b Pair Work Practice with another student. Give answers following the model at left.

2 a Match the questions and answers.

Questions
1 You weren't really late for the interview, were you?
2 They've always had leadership potential, haven't they?
3 You should have said you'd be away tomorrow, shouldn't you?
4 They haven't gotten used to your style already, have they?
5 Yes, it was a tough interview, but it was also a valuable experience, wasn't it?

Answers
.... I did. Unfortunately, the message got lost in the system.
.... Yes. Everything I do seems predictable these days.
.... Yes. I learned a lot from it, I guess.
.... Only a few minutes, but they weren't ready for me, anyway.
.... No. It's something they developed during the training program.

b Pair Work Think of your own answers, and practice asking and answering the questions with a partner.

3 Complete the following statements with appropriate tags.

1 "You should have called, ... ?"
2 "You've been a group leader before, ... ?"
3 "You've never considered yourself more of a follower than a leader, ... ?"
4 "Most of the students in the class seem self-motivated, ... ?"
5 "Most people have a healthy attitude towards people from other cultures, ... ?"
6 "We'd all rather cooperate than compete, ... ?

---

1. **(a)** This task involves students in actively thinking about how English works. Rather than simply being given the grammar rule, students are encouraged to study the examples—to recognize language patterns and figure out grammar/language rules for themselves. (Answers: 1—yes; 2—no; 3—no; 4—yes; 5—yes; 6—yes)

(b) Have students work in pairs to ask and answer questions, using the sample language as a model.

Do you know the rule? (Answers: positive answer—negative tag; negative answer—positive tag)

2. **(a)** Working individually, students complete the statements, following the previous examples. Circulate and offer help when necessary. (Answers: 1—Only a few minutes; 2—No. It's something they developed; 3—I did . . . the message got lost; 4—Yes. Everything . . . predictable; 5—Yes. I learned a lot)

(b) Students think of new answers to the questions and then practice asking and answering with a partner.

3. Students provide the appropriate tag questions. (Suggested answers: 1—shouldn't you; 2—have you; 3—have you; 4—don't they; 5—don't you think; 6—wouldn't we)

Self-Check

Communication Challenge

Challenge 12 is on pages 122 and 124 of the student text, and suggestions for its use are on page 122 in this Teacher's Extended Edition.

1. Encourage students to complete this task without looking back at the unit.

2. In groups of at least three, students brainstorm ideas about when/where they might speculate about the future and check and confirm facts and opinions. Circulate and make sure the suggestions are as specific as possible. Encourage students to think about situations they have been in when they needed to use this language. Elicit responses from the class.

3. Before students carry out the survey, give them time to decide who they will ask and exactly how they will ask their questions. Have students draw up a survey sheet on which they will record both positive and negative answers. After the surveys, students report to the class the information they gathered. List on the board all qualities those surveyed considered positive and all those they disliked. With the whole class, discuss the responses.

4. Have students work individually to check off the words that they know.

• The grammar summary for this unit is on page 133.

Self-Check

COMMUNICATION CHALLENGE

PairWork Student A: Look at Challenge 12A on page 122. Student B: Look at Challenge 12B on page 124.

1 Write three new sentences or questions you learned.

2 Review the language skills you practiced in this unit. In what situations might you use this language?

WHEN WOULD YOU USE THIS LANGUAGE?

	Situations
Speculate about future actions	
Check and confirm facts and opinions	

3 Out of Class Talk to a friend or relative about the people they work with or go to school with. Make a list of the qualities they admire and dislike in other people. Report back to the class and make a single list. What similarities/differences are there in what people reported?

GOOD QUALITIES	BAD QUALITIES

4 Vocabulary check. Check [√] the words you know.

Adjectives/Adverbs
- caring
- challenging
- consistent
- constructive
- detailed
- dynamic
- hopeful
- limited
- multicultural
- negative
- optimistic
- particularly
- pessimistic
- potential
- prepared
- talented
- upbeat

Nouns
- applicant
- attitude
- authority
- conditions
- creativity
- economy
- equal opportunity
- evaluation
- hope
- job opportunity
- knowledge
- leadership
- optimist
- orchestra
- organization
- pessimist
- principal
- strength
- talent

Verbs
- agree
- delegate
- demonstrate
- disagree
- extend
- speculate

13 Time For a Change

Warm-Up

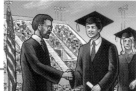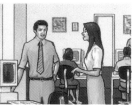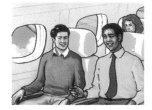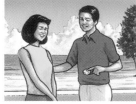

Unit Goals

In this unit you will:

Express past and future expectations

"We were supposed to have gone to Yani's party last weekend."

"I'm supposed to sign up for the new aerobics class by Friday."

Describe interesting and significant events in the past

"Well, I spent a year in Brazil as an exchange student."

1 Look at the person in the pictures. What significant events are occurring in his life?

2 a **Group Work** Discussion. Talk about significant things that have happened to you in these categories:

- education
- travel
- employment
- relationships

b **Group Work** In what ways did these events change your life?

c **Group Work** What things do you expect to happen to you in the next few years in these areas of your life?

3 a **Group Work** Discussion. Do you . . .

- get up at the same time every day?
- have the same thing for breakfast every day?
- hang out with the same people most of the time?
- watch the same shows on television every week?
- wear the same kind of clothing most of the time?
- do the same kinds of exercise all the time?

b **Group Work** Compare your responses with three or four other students. How predictable are you? Who is the most/least predictable person in the group?

Warm-Up

Unit Goals. This section presents the language of expressing past and future expectations, and describing interesting and significant events in the past. Choose individual students to read out each of the goals and the examples, or read them yourself. Have students circle the ones that they feel they can do in English.

1. Working individually, students identify the events shown in the pictures. Elicit responses from around the class.
(Answers will vary.)

2. (a) Give students time to consider these four areas of life and at least one significant thing that has happened to them in each of the areas. You may want to ask students to think about this outside class, before the lesson. Then have students discuss their answers in groups.

(b) New learning is successful only if it has personal relevance and meaning for learners. Have students work in groups to talk over the implications of the events they discussed in (a).

(c) Speculating or predicting is an important thinking skill and an important strategy in successful communication. This task gives students the opportunity to speculate from their own knowledge and experience and discuss their speculations with their group. Circulate and monitor content and pronunciation.

3. (a) Give students one or two examples from your own daily routine as a model. Then have students work in groups to answer the questions. Provide help as necessary.

(b) In small groups, students compare and discuss their responses. **Variation.** Have students extend the discussion to include the advantages or disadvantages of doing the same things every day or every week.

Task Chain 1: Changing times

Task 1. (a) In pairs, students note any differences between the pictures and match the pictures to a time period.
(Answers will vary.)

Variation. With the whole class, discuss what details help us identify periods from past eras. What are some obvious visual features or characteristics of our own time?

(b) Encourage students to prepare for this task by talking to any relatives or friends who can remember life 30 or 40 years ago. Ask students to think about the major changes experienced by the people in the first two pictures as they grew up. Also get them to think about what major changes might be experienced in the next 20 years by the children in the third picture.
(Answers will vary.)

(c) This task enables students to use their imagination to speculate. Remind them that speculating, like predicting, is not random, but a well-defined learning strategy in which students use their existing knowledge and experience to make informed and intelligent guesses.
(Answers will vary.)

Learning Strategy. All listening is selective. We listen for what is important or interesting to us, and we filter out the rest. It is very important to practice tasks that help to develop the skill of listening in this way.

Task Chain 1 Changing times

Task 1

a Pair Work Look at the pictures. When do you think they were taken? What differences do you see among the pictures?

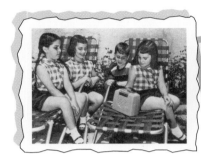 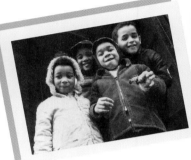 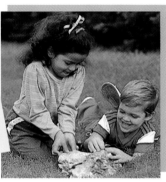

Picture 1   Picture 2   Picture 3

b What do you think were the major changes experienced by the people in the first two pictures as they grew up? Make notes in the blank lines below. Over the next 20 years, what do you think will be the major changes experienced by the children in the third picture?

Picture 1 ....

....

Picture 2 ....

....

Picture 3 ....

....

"Forty years ago, many children didn't finish high school. Most children born today can probably expect to go to college."

LEARNING STRATEGY

Selective listening = listening for the most important words and information.

c What did children born forty years ago expect for their future? What do children born now expect? What differences do you think there are? Make notes in the chart and discuss your ideas.

	40 YEARS AGO	NOW
education		
health		
employment		
leisure		

Task 2

a 🎧 Listen. You will hear two of the people in the pictures from Task 1 talking about their lives. Try to guess when each speaker was born and what they are talking about.

Speaker 1 was born .... years ago. Topic: ....

Speaker 2 was born .... years ago. Topic: ....

b 🎧 Listen again to the first speaker and list all the differences he notes between his life as a young adult and his life now.

Then	*Now*
....	....
....	....
....	....
....	....
....	....

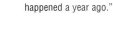

"Well, the most significant event was meeting her boyfriend—that happened a year ago."

c 🎧 Listen again to the second speaker and note the significant events.

Event	*When*
1	....
2	....
3	....
4	....
5	....

d **Group Work** Work with two other students to decide when these events occurred.

Task 3

a What are the differences between your life now and 5, 10, and 15 years ago? Fill in the chart.

"Well, fifteen years ago, I was a child living at home and totally dependent on my parents. Today, I share an apartment with my brother. Ten years ago, I was just starting high school, whereas today I have a college diploma."

	5 YEARS AGO	**10 YEARS AGO**	**15 YEARS AGO**
work			
relationships			
living arrangements			
education			

b **Group Work** Discuss your responses.

Task 2. **(a)** 🎧 Do this task in two stages. Play the tape once. Have students listen for who the people are and how old they seem to be. Play the tape again, and this time have students listen for what the speakers are speaking about. Let students take notes as they listen. (Suggested answers: Speaker 1—forty to fifty; life changes. Speaker 2—approximately twenty-five; important events.)

(b) 🎧 Play the tape again. It is very important for language learners to develop skills in listening for key information. In this task they listen selectively for the differences between the speaker's life as a young man and his life now.
(Answers: Then—rode motorcycle to work; Now—drives car. Then—shared small apartment with three other young men and ate poorly; Now—lives in decent house and is able to eat out. Then—went surfing down the coast. Now—goes to a resort in Florida and plays golf. Then—just married; Now—recently divorced.)

(c, d) 🎧 Play the tape once more. Have students listen and fill out the first column of the chart with the information about events in the second speaker's life. Then have students work in groups to determine when these events happened and fill out the second column of the chart.
(Answers: new boyfriend/about a year ago; marriage proposal/last week; spending a year in Brazil/age fifteen; going to community college/age eighteen; getting a new job/last month)

Task 3. **(a)** Learning tasks are more successful when learners have a specific focus. Have learners think about where they were living and what they were doing 5, 10, 15 years ago. They then think of the most important or significant thing that happened to them at that time. Each student completes the table as an individual writing task. Circulate and check spelling.

(b) In small groups, students compare and discuss their completed tables.

Language Focus 1: Review of past & perfect tenses

1. **(a)** Give students time to read through the letter at least twice. Then have them provide the correct verb tense for the seven verbs.
(Answers: 1—have been having; 2—have grown up; 3—came; 4—had been; 5—was playing; 6—am seeing; 7—was talking)

(b) Have students fill out the chart by listing the verb numbers from the letter in the appropriate columns.
(Answers: simple past—3; present perfect—1, 2; past perfect—4; present perfect progressive—6; past perfect progressive—5, 7)

2. **(a)** Have students do this as an individual writing task. Circulate and monitor grammar and spelling.

(b) After students have come up with their three questions, give them time to practice them so that they can interview their classmates without referring to their notes.

3. **(a)** Guide this task by brainstorming with the whole class which stages in their life they might consider—childhood, school days, teenage years, their first jobs—and what kinds of events—accidents, loss, discovery, success, failure, birth, death. Then have each student make notes on one event from his or her life, using as many past and perfect tense forms as possible.

(b) Each student retells their story to a small group while the others note the verb tenses used.

Language Focus 1 Review of past & perfect tenses

Dear Deb,

Please help me. I (1) .... (have) terrible problems with my parents recently. They just don't understand me. I'm almost an adult, but they simply don't seem to realize that I (2) .... (grow up), and they continue to treat me as though I were a child. I've never been allowed to stay out after nine o'clock at night. Last week I (3) .... (come) in at nine thirty, and they said that I wasn't allowed out for the next month because they (4) .... (be) so worried. I (5) .... (play) cards at my friend's house next door. Now, the big problem is that I (6) .... (see) this guy at school for a few months. My parents don't know of course—they wouldn't approve, but I really like him. Anyway, I (7) .... (talk) with him on the phone the other day, and he asked me to come to his parents' anniversary party next Saturday night. But I can't go because I'm grounded! What should I do?

1 **a** Read the following letter and put the verbs in parentheses into the appropriate tense.

b Identify the tenses in the blanks by writing the number in the chart.

TENSE	BLANK
simple past	
present perfect	
past perfect	
present perfect progressive	
past perfect progressive	

"I studied Portuguese for two years before learning English."

2 **a** Answer the following questions, giving as many details as you can.

1 When did you first use English outside of the classroom?
....

2 Has anyone ever spoken to you in English outside of the classroom?
....

3 How long have you been learning English?
....

4 Had you studied any other languages before learning English?
....

b Now think of three additional questions and interview two other students.

1 .... ?
2 .... ?
3 .... ?

3 **a** Think of some dramatic or important event in your life. Make notes using as many of the past and perfect tense forms as you can.

b **GroupWork** Take turns telling your story. Your partners will note the different tense forms they hear.

Task Chain 2 Get out of that rut!

"Well, I'll definitely reduce the amount of TV I watch. I might try changing my workout. But I would definitely never take a healthful vacation."

Task 1

a 🎧 **Group Work** Listen. What is wrong with Barbara? What does her friend offer to do? What do you think being in a "rut" means?

b **Group Work** Are you in a rut? Brainstorm ways of changing your daily routine.

Task 2

a Skim the following article and add these subheadings in the blanks:

Personal Development   **Career Changes**   **At Leisure**
Family and Community   **Better Health**

b Read the article again and decide which of these things you will definitely/might/would never do to get out of a rut.

c **Group Work** Discuss your responses with three or four other students.

The Same Old Life: Getting Yourself Out of a Rut

You've eaten the same thing for breakfast every day for three years, then taken the same car pool to the same job. Your life is more of the same after work. It's time to get out of your rut. Making any of the following small changes can lead to big changes in your life.

- Learn a new job skill. Pick something you have always wanted to do, such as learning a new computer program. Take a class at a community college.
- Earn that college degree. Study a course catalog to determine what it takes to get started. Or earn a certificate given by the professional association in your field. Inform your supervisor about your goal.
- Subscribe to a professional or career journal in your field. If you already subscribe to one, write an article or letter to the editor.

- Reduce the amount of time you spend watching television by an hour a day. Use the extra time for something special, such as reading a book or doing a hobby.
- Start a family project, such as planning your next vacation or planting a backyard garden.
- Fulfill a fantasy. For example, take dancing lessons, or join a neighborhood chess club or sports team.

- Take a walk. Use your lunch break to explore the neighborhood near your workplace.
- Vary your workout. Add new challenges by making your workout more interesting.
- Explore a new cuisine. Sample local ethnic restaurants or learn to make new dishes.
- Take a healthful vacation. Attend a sports camp or sign up for a bike tour of a national park.

- Play "tourist" in your own town. Check out a guidebook or ask your visitor's bureau for information on local tourist attractions.
- Take your camera with you on daily activities. Look for scenes that would make interesting pictures.
- Write a letter to someone you haven't heard from in a while. It might revive a friendship.

- Ask your children, spouse, or friends to suggest their favorite things to do, then join in—enthusiastically.
- Volunteer. A nearby hospital, library, or theater group could probably use your help. Start by committing yourself to a single event or project. If you enjoy the work, you can build a long-term relationship.

Source: *Vitality*, June 1994.

Task Chain 2: Get out of that rut!

Task 1. (a) 🎧 Discuss with the class the strategy of deducing meaning from context. Students often stop listening when they hear a word they do not know, but continuing to listen can help them guess the meaning of the new word from other information in the text. Play the tape. From context, students answer the questions and give opinions about what *being in a rut* means. Elicit answers from each group.
(Answers: She's in a rut. Her friend offers to show her a newspaper article about ways of getting out of a rut.)

(b) Give students time to look back at their answers to Warm-Up Task 3 and think of things they would like to change. Then, in groups, they discuss and compare their responses. For the second part of this task, give students time to brainstorm ways to get out of daily ruts and routines.

Task 2. (a) Read the subheadings with the whole class, and explain any that students do not understand. Remind students of the reading strategy of skimming for specific information. Students then read the article at least twice, marking key words or phrases that help them match the subheading to its section. Circulate and provide assistance if necessary. **Variation.** Students do this in groups, discussing their views and reaching a consensus about where each subheading belongs.
(Answers, in order: Career Changes; Personal Development; Better Health; At Leisure; Family and Community)

(b) Working individually, students read the article again and decide which suggestions they would or would not use to help them change their routine. Have students practice expressing their opinion, using the sample language as a model. Circulate and monitor pronunciation.

(c) In groups, students compare their responses and practice saying them to one another.

Task 3. **(a)** In pairs, students create a written survey from the information in the article. Have them read the article again and select information from under each subheading to translate into questions. Circulate and provide help as necessary. Have students write out their questions, in full or in note form, and then practice asking them so that they can avoid referring to their written notes. Monitor pronunciation and grammar.

(b) Each student surveys three others in the class and notes their responses on the survey sheet. Then, in pairs, students compare the responses they got.

Task 4. 🎧 Do this listening task in two stages. Play the tape once, and have students listen for and write down the new things that Barbara tried. Then play the tape again, and this time students listen for what happened to her each time she tried something new. (Answers: Career—to learn TypeRight; couldn't enroll in class. Personal development—to take an art class; art supplies too expensive. Health—to take up jogging; twisted her ankle. Leisure—to play tourist in her own town; it rained all day. Family/community—to volunteer at a library; needed librarian training.)

Task 5. **(a)** Remind students of the importance of linking the learning to their own lives and opinions. With the whole class, brainstorm areas of life that students might consider changing. Have students fill out the first column of the chart.

(b) Encourage each student to think about and write down specific changes that he or she would like to make in one or more of these areas. Have students work in pairs to plan specific changes. Monitor the language they use to express their opinions.

(c) Combine pairs, and have students compare and discuss their plans. Make this a speaking practice task. Circulate and check pronunciation.

	STUDENT 1 yes maybe no	STUDENT 2 yes maybe no	STUDENT 3 yes maybe no
Learn a new job skill	☐ ☐	☐ ☐	☐ ☐

A If you were in a rut, would you learn a new job skill?

B You must be kidding—change one rut for another?

A I'd like to make some new friends.

B Why don't you join a club?

Task 3

a Pair Work Create a survey to find out how other students would get out of a rut. Add your own ideas or use the suggestions from the article.

b Group Work Interview three other students to find out if they would use these ideas to get out of a rut. Now compare results with your partner.

Task 4

🎧 In Task 1, you heard Barbara talking about being in a rut. Her friend gave her a copy of the article from Task 2, and is now asking her about what changes she made. Listen to the plans she made, and the results. Make notes in the chart

	PLAN	RESULT
Career		
Personal development		
Health		
Leisure		
Family/community		

Task 5

a Think of three things about your lifestyle that you would like to change and write them in the first column.

WHAT I PLAN TO CHANGE	HOW I PLAN TO CHANGE
1	
2	
3	

b Pair Work Work together to make a plan to change. Write your plans in the second column.

c Group Work Compare plans with another pair.

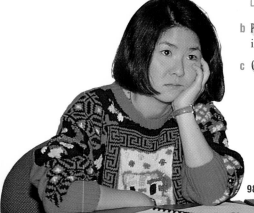

Language Focus 2 *Supposed to*

1 Which of the following refer to past events and which to future events? Write P for past events and F for future expectations in the blank next to each sentence.

.... I'm supposed to enroll in the new computer course by Friday.

.... They were supposed to have sent me the enrollment form in the mail.

.... We were supposed to have completed the assignment by the end of semester.

.... The survey is supposed to be published by the end of the week.

.... The interviewer was supposed to have asked more detailed questions.

.... They are supposed to provide the information in time for next weekend's newspapers.

2 Complete the following statements.

a Barbara was supposed to have learned a new wordprocessing program, but ....

b She was supposed to have taken up painting, but ....
....

c She .... , but she twisted her ankle.

d She was supposed to have taken a tour of the city, but ....
....

e She .... , but she had no librarian training.

3 a Think of ways to complete these statements.

1 The teacher was supposed to have given us an exam yesterday, but ....

2 We were supposed to have prepared for the exam, but ....

3 They are supposed to come to the party, but ....

4 We are supposed to finish the assignment by Monday, but ....

5 The teacher was supposed to have handed our last assignment back to us by Friday, but ....

b **Group Work** Compare responses. Who has the most interesting or unusual responses?

"Adriana was supposed to have called her parents last week, but she forgot."

4 a **Pair Work** Find out three things that your partner was supposed to have done in the last month, but didn't do.

b **Group Work** Report what your partner said to another pair.

c **Pair Work** Write down three things you are supposed to do by the end of the year and then tell another student.

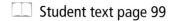 Student text page 99

Language Focus 2: *Supposed to*

1. Have each student read through the sentences and mark the verbs in each one. Then students decide whether the sentence is about the past or about the future. Elicit answers from around the class. (Answers: future; past; past; future; past; future)

2. In this task students supply their own language from the models and examples they have been working with. Give them several minutes to consider the task—that is, what they will say to complete the statement and how they will say it. Circulate and check content, spelling, and grammar. Have individual students read their statements to the class. **Optional.** In pairs, students compare their answers and choose only one for each sentence. (Answers will vary.)

3. (**a**) Give students several minutes to read the beginnings of the statements and consider how they might finish them. Then have them complete the statements. Circulate and correct content, spelling, and grammar before students write their final versions, which should incorporate your corrections.

(**b**) Have groups of students read, compare, and discuss their statements. Have the group vote on the most interesting or unusual responses.

4. (**a**) Remind the class that *supposed to* refers to something that did not get done. Give students time to think about three things they should have done in the last month but did not. Then, in pairs, students survey their partner and write down their responses. Allow them to write notes rather than complete sentences if they so desire.

(**b**) Combine two pairs and have each student report to the group what his or her partner said, using the sample language as a model.

(**c**) Give students time to think about three things they are supposed to have done by the end of the year. They then write these and read them to a partner. Circulate and monitor spelling, grammar, and content.

Self-Check

Communication Challenge

Challenge 13 is on page 126 of the student text, and suggestions for its use are on that page in this Teacher's Extended Edition.

1. Encourage students to complete this task without looking back at the unit.

2. **(a)** Students think about when and where they might express expectations and narrate a sequence of events from the past. Make sure that students are as specific as possible. Encourage them to think about situations they have been in when they needed to use this language. **Optional.** In class, students compare responses. Elicit responses from the class.

   (b) Have two or three students work together to brainstorm ideas about where and when they could practice expressing their expectations and narrating a sequence of events. You may want to have them do this out of class and then report their ideas back to the whole class at the next lesson.

3. Retelling events or anecdotes is an important language skill. Encourage students to ask the person to tell the story at least twice. Students should make notes as they listen to the story.

4. Have students work individually to check off the words that they know.

• The grammar summary for this unit is on page 134.

Self-Check

COMMUNICATION CHALLENGE

GroupWork Look at Challenge 13 on page 126.

1 Write three new sentences or questions you learned.

....

....

....

2 a Review the language skills you practiced in this unit. In what situations might you use this language?

WHEN WOULD YOU USE THIS LANGUAGE?

	Situations
Express past and future expectations	
Describe interesting and significant events in the past	

b **GroupWork** Brainstorm ways to practice this language out of class. Imagine you are visiting an English-speaking country. Where/When might you need this language?

3 **Out of Class** Find someone who has an interesting or dramatic story to tell. Make notes, and then retell the story in class. Who has the most interesting or most dramatic story?

Name	Story Events
1.	
2.	

4 Vocabulary check. Check [√] the words you know.

Adjectives/Adverbs			Nouns			Verbs		
☐ dependent	☐ main	☐ significant	☐ catalog	☐ expectations	☐ supervisor	☐ approve	☐ happen	☐ sample
☐ ethnic	☐ predictable	☐ totally	☐ car pool	☐ leisure	☐ workout	☐ break out	☐ help	☐ subscribe
☐ ever	☐ professional		☐ change	☐ relationships		☐ change	☐ note	☐ understand
☐ first	☐ selective		☐ difference	☐ rut		☐ experience	☐ occur	☐ vary

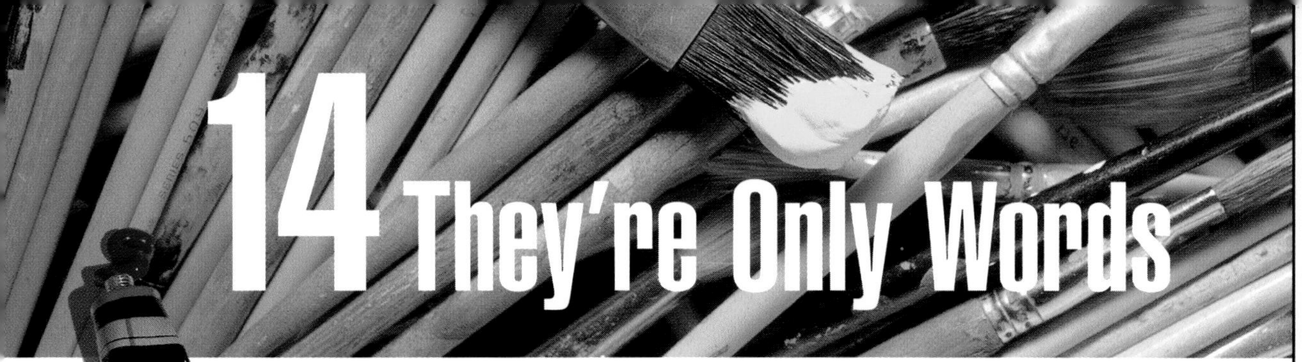

14 They're Only Words

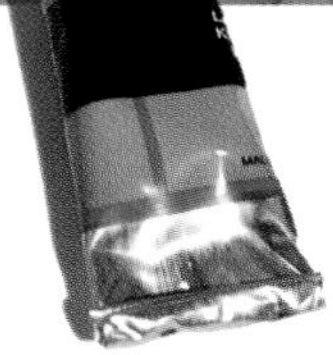

Warm-Up

Unit Goals

In this unit you will:

Talk about cultural attitudes and beliefs

"In some cultures, it is considered unlucky to keep certain kinds of animals as pets."

Express a point of view

"People who paint graffiti are destructive vandals who ought to be punished."

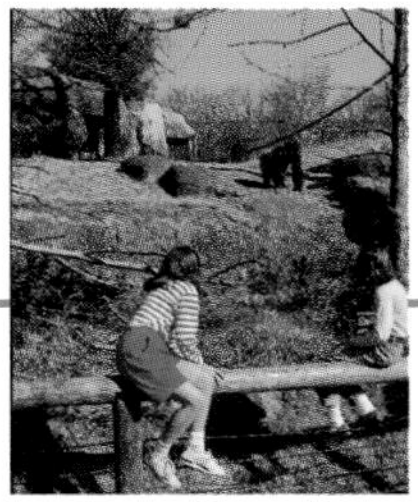

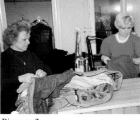
Picture 1

Picture 2

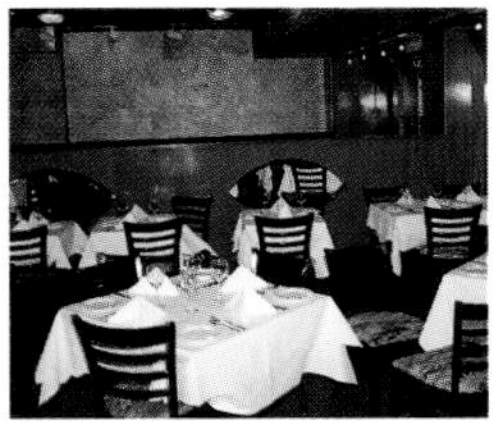

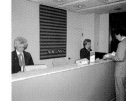
Picture 3

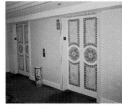
Picture 4

Picture 5

1 Look at the pictures. Where would you see these notices? Write the number of the picture in the correct blank.

....

Customers may have a fit upstairs.

....

Our wines leave nothing to hope for.

....

Guests are expected to complain to the manager between the hours of 9 and 11 A.M. daily.

....

Please do not feed the animals. If you have food, please give it to the guard on duty.

....

We take your bags and send them in all directions.

2 What is wrong with the notices? Correct them.

📖 Student text page 101

Warm-Up

Unit Goals. This section presents the language of talking about cultural attitudes and beliefs and expressing a point of view. Choose individual students to read aloud each of the goals and the examples, or read them yourself. Have students circle those that they feel they can do in English.

1. Have students examine the pictures and match the notices to them.
(Answers: Picture 1—Please do not feed the animals. Picture 2—Guests are expected to complain. Picture 3—Our wines leave nothing to hope for. Picture 4—We take your bags and send them in all directions. Picture 5—Customers may have a fit upstairs.)

2. Read the sentences through, once, with the whole class, without any discussion. Then have students find the errors and correct them.
(Suggested answers: Customers may have a *fitting* upstairs. Our wines leave nothing to *wish* for. We take your bags and send them *wherever you are going*. If you have food, the guard on duty *can dispose of it*. The manager *can handle complaints* between the hours of 9 and 11 a.m. daily.)

Task Chain 1: The magic of language

Task 1. (a) With the whole class, discuss the kind of information given about a word in the dictionary: meaning, pronunciation, related words, origin of the word, part of speech. List these on the board. Give students time to read through the two word meanings at least twice. Explain any abbreviations that students do not know. Then have students work in pairs to discuss what they think the words have in common.

(b) If there are speakers of different languages in the class, group together people who speak the same language. If all students have the same first language, group them randomly. Students then discuss the three questions. Manage the discussion so that the most talkative students do not dominate. Call on one member of each group to report the group's answers to the whole class. **Variation.** Have students prepare for the discussion outside class, before the lesson, and, if possible, talk about the questions with other speakers of their language.

Task 2. (a, b) 🎧 Play the tape. Students listen and write down any taboos that are mentioned, completing the first column of the chart. Then play the tape again so that students can listen for the societies in which these taboos exist.
(Answers: supernatural, sex, death—many societies; use of word "frog"—Zuni Indians in New Mexico; use of word "bull"—United States; individuals' names—Aborigines in Australia)

(c) Students consider euphemisms for death used in the different societies discussed in the conversation. Elicit answers from around the class.

(d) Have students work in pairs to come up with new questions for the interviewer to ask the anthropologist. Have them practice asking and answering questions.

Task Chain 1 The magic of language

Task 1

a **Pair Work** Discussion. In this chain you will use the words *taboo* and *euphemism*. Look at these definitions and decide what the words have in common.

> **taboo** *n.* **1** an act or subject that religion or society dissaproves of strongly: *There is a taboo against couples living together before marriage in many societies.* **2** an agreement not to discuss (touch, do, etc.) s.t. *-adj.* under a taboo: *It is taboo to use bad words in front of my parents.*
>
> **euphemism** *n.* **1** a more pleasant word or description used to replace a word or description that is considered unpleasant: *To say, "heavy" is a euphemism for "fat". -adj.* **euphemistic.**

From *The Newbury House Dictionary of American English.*

b Does your language have taboo words or euphemisms? What happens when people use these words? Have some taboo words become more acceptable in recent years?

Task 2

a 🎧 Listen to the anthropologist talking about taboos in different societies. What taboos are mentioned? Listen and fill in the blanks under "taboo".

TABOO	SOCIETY
supernatural, sex, death	
	Zuni Indians in New Mexico
use of word "bull"	
	Aborigines in Australia

b 🎧 Now listen again for the societies where these things are taboo. Fill in the blanks under "society".

c What are some of the euphemisms for *death*?

d **Pair Work** Imagine you are the interviewer. What questions would you like to ask the anthropologist?

Task 3

a Pair Work Discussion. Skim the following text. How would you describe the tone? Check [√] one.

☐ humorous   ☐ serious   ☐ sarcastic   ☐ academic

Have you noticed how the English language is changing from under our very tongues? We don't throw trash out of our homes any more but dispose of "recyclable products." This obsession for creating euphemisms is even extending to the world of employment.

The other day, *The Southern Express* ran an advertisement for a firm looking for a Leathergoods Maintenance Officer: Footwear Division. What on earth would such a person do? Why, shine shoes, of course. Because the term "shoeshine boy" is no longer politically correct (and who wants to shine shoes anyway, even one's own?), the person who wrote the advertisement came up with a nice euphemism. Of course, the person who gets the job will still end up shining shoes.

The same firm is also looking for a Sanitary Engineer: Personnel Services. Such a person used to be called a Washroom Attendant, someone who hands out towels and cleans up the messy public washroom. However, providing a personal service is much more dignified than attending to other people's messy habits.

And employers aren't the only ones who are experts at creating euphemisms. Recently, one well-known journalist was accused of lying. He denied the accusation, but admitted that he might have been economical with the truth. A politician accused of being drunk at a public function also denied the charge, saying that he had been tired and emotional.

What do these examples tell us? Well, they either indicate that as a language English is alive and well, or that it is about to pass away.

ORIGINAL TERM	EUPHEMISM
to lie	
trash	
to be drunk	

b What euphemisms does the article use for the following terms?

c Which professions does the article name as using euphemisms?

Task 4

a Pair Work What do you think the following expressions mean?

"to pass away" ....
"to carry a few extra pounds" ....
"to have a preowned car" ....
"to be temporarily embarrassed for money" ....
"to depart from the truth" ....

b Group Work Compare your responses with another pair's responses.

c Pair Work Think of euphemisms for the following jobs and compare your euphemism with another person.

Cleaner   Street-corner vendor   Hotel doorperson
Waiter   Security guard

"Well, we think that 'to pass away' means 'to die'."

Task 3.   (a) Before the reading, discuss with the whole class the meaning of each of the describing words—*humorous, serious, sarcastic,* and *academic*. In pairs, students read the article and decide which of the words best describes the tone of the text.
(Answer: *humorous* is the best choice, but a case can be made for *sarcastic*.)

(b) Remind students of what a euphemism is: a mild, indirect, or vague expression used in place of a direct or blunt one. Sometimes euphemisms exaggerate the positive perspective or obscure the real meaning too much and can be misleading. Have each student reread the article and fill out the chart.
(Answers: to lie—being economical with the truth; trash—recyclable products; to be drunk—tired and emotional)

(c) Have students read through the article again and note which professions are named as using euphemisms. Elicit responses from around the class.
(Answers will vary in wording but should reflect the information in the article.)

Task 4.   (a) Discuss with the class the strategy of deducing meaning from context. Then, in pairs, students deduce or make intelligent guesses about the meanings of these expressions.
(Answers: to die; to be fat; to have a used car; to be broke; to lie)

(b) Combine pairs and have students compare and discuss their opinions. Make sure they practice speaking, using the sample language as a model.

(c) Have students work individually to come up with euphemisms for the jobs and then compare their responses with a partner.

Language Focus 1: Complex passives

1. **(a)** This is a language-creating task in which students combine parts of sentences to form a complete statement. Have students do this as an individual writing task.
(Answers: 1. In our super-sophisticated society, it is believed that certain subjects are unlucky. 2. In many different societies, it is considered unlucky to mention animal names. 3. Among some Australian aboriginal tribes, it is believed that a person's name should never be used. 4. Among the Zuni Indians of New Mexico, it is prohibited to use the word for "frogs." 5. In parts of the United States, it is considered improper to use the word "bull.")
(b) 🎧 Play the tape at least twice so that students can check their responses.

2. Have students work in pairs. Circulate and provide assistance where necessary. With the whole class, go through the list and check answers.
(Suggested answers: a—In some places, it is believed that words have magic properties. b—In some Australian aboriginal tribes, it is prohibited to use people's private names. c—In ancient times, it was thought that language could cure sickness and disease. d—Sometimes, it is assumed that changing the name of a place will bring good luck.)

3. **(a)** Allow time for students to practice and become familiar with what they will say so that they refer to the written form as little as possible. Then students work in pairs to practice asking and answering the questions. Monitor and correct content, grammar, and pronunciation.
(b) Students swap roles and practice again.

4. Have students work in groups to practice making statements about taboos in their country. Make sure that they use the sample language as a model.

Language Focus 1 Complex passives

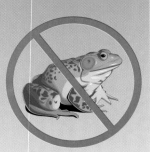

1 a Match column 1 with column 2 to complete the statements.

Column 1
1 In our super-sophisticated society,
2 In many different societies,
3 Among some Australian aboriginal tribes,
4 Among the Zuni Indians of New Mexico,
5 In parts of the United States,

Column 2
.... it is believed that a person's name should never be used.
.... it is considered unlucky to mention animal names.
.... it is considered improper to use the word "bull".
.... it is believed that certain subjects are unlucky.
.... it is prohibited to use the word for "frogs".

b 🎧 Listen to the tape and check your answers.

2 **Pair Work** Make statements following the model at left.

a In some places, people believe that words have magic properties.
b In some Australian aboriginal tribes, members have public and private names.
c In ancient times, people thought that language could cure sickness and disease.
d People sometimes assume that changing the name of a place will bring good luck.

3 a **Pair Work** Student A plays the part of an interviewer. Student B plays the part of a famous anthropologist. Ask and answer questions using these cues.

A: Are taboos only found in primitive societies?
B: No / sophisticated societies / believed / certain subjects are unlucky
A: Can you give examples of animal taboos?
B: New Mexico / believed / bad / mention / word for frogs
A: What is the most extraordinary taboo you know of?
B: Among Australian Aborigines / prohibited for / person's name / be mentioned
A: What happens if taboos are broken?
B: in many societies / not unusual / people / be severely punished

b Now change roles and do the task again.

4 **Group Work** Think of three taboos in your country. Take turns making statements about them, using the model at left.

"In most societies, people believe it is unlucky to talk about death."

"In most societies, it is believed unlucky to talk about death."

"In our society, it is considered a taboo to mention . . ."

Task 1

a 🎧 You will hear a disagreement between two people. They are arguing over an incident that was reported in the newspaper with this headline. Can you predict what the argument is about?

The Town Crier

Four-Month Suspended Sentence for Spray-Can Kid

b 🎧 Listen and make a note of the arguments for and against the graffiti artist.

ARGUMENTS FOR	ARGUMENTS AGAINST

c Which of the pieces of graffiti pictured did Dennis Wilson paint?

Picture 1

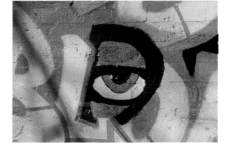

Picture 2

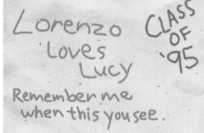

Lorenzo CLASS OF Loves Lucy '95

Remember me when this you see.

Task Chain 2: Playing with words

Task 1. (a) 🎧 Predicting allows students to exchange ideas freely and also prepares them for what they will hear. Play the tape, and after the conversation has concluded, ask students if their predictions were correct.

(b) 🎧 Play the tape again. Students listen for the main points of the argument and fill out the chart. (Suggested answers: For—not graffiti but attractive art; Dennis painted an ugly wall; Dennis has talent but few outlets with which to express himself. Against—he destroyed public property; he shows a lack of respect for traditional values; he created ugly, modern art; taxpayer money will have to be used to remove the graffiti.)

(c) Students examine the graffiti. They decide which example was painted by Dennis Wilson. (Answer: Picture 2)

Task 2. (a) In this task students read for specific information. Give them sufficient time to read through the letters at least twice. They decide which of the letters are sympathetic to the graffiti artist and which are not. Have them underline words and phrases that show the writer's point of view.
(Answers: Letter 1—against; Letter 2—for; Letter 3—for; Letter 4—against)

(b) Have students consider which of the letters might have been written by one of the speakers in Task 1. Make sure that students give reasons to support their opinions.
(Answer: Letter 3)

(c) Do this as an individual writing task. Allow students time to write two drafts. After they have completed the first draft, they should correct and revise it, with your help or by helping each other. They then write a second draft that incorporates any corrections or changes.

Task 3. (a) Each pair decides which opinion about Dennis that each partner will argue. Then give them enough time to consider what they will say and how they will express it, using the sample language as a model.

(b) Students change partners and roles and go through the process again. Remind them that this is a speaking task. Circulate and monitor pronunciation.

Learning Strategy. Sharing ideas and experiences with others can help us to understand better how we think and how we learn. Group and pair work, in class, provide excellent opportunities for learning how others think and comparing different ways of learning.

Task 4. (a) With the whole class, review this structure: "If I came across someone spraying graffiti, I would. . . . Encourage students to think about a specific situation—that is, the place, the time of day, what they are doing, whether they are alone or not. Give them time to consider what they would do in this situation. They then discuss this in their group.

(b) Combine two groups and have them compare and discuss what they would do.

Letter 1

Dear Madam,

I write to express my disgust at the rather weak-minded attitude taken by your newspaper towards the sentence given to a certain Dennis Wilson. We expect the press to uphold the law, not to undermine it. I do not know the young man, but I believe he has been in trouble more than once before. Perhaps this will teach him a lesson he won't forget.

Letter 2

Dear Editor,

I was encouraged by the attitude taken by your newspaper on the matter of young Dennis Wilson. Far from being the menace that some people say he is, Dennis is a responsible, though high-spirited youth who is well known in the neighborhood. As he said to the judge, he was only trying to brighten up the neighborhood with a "mural". I must say that I enjoy looking at the mural as I walk to work in the morning.

Letter 3

To the Editor:

I was disappointed at the harsh and unfair reactions of much of the community in the case of Dennis Wilson. The boy is creative and gifted, and the work of art which he has produced is a major improvement to what was an ugly wall. To call it graffiti is absurd. It might look a little strange to those people who do not appreciate modern art, but surely even they would rather look at a colorful wall than a dirty concrete one. I believe that the judge in this case made a mistake, and I would like to take this opportunity of congratulating you for pointing this out.

Letter 4

Editor:

I wish to cancel my subscription to your newspaper. The attitude you took to the Wilson case has totally destroyed your credibility as far as I am concerned. Your role is to report the facts objectively, not to express opinions. As far as I am concerned, that boy got off too lightly. He's a menace to himself and all of those around him.

Task 2

a Here are some letters to the local paper about the Wilson incident. Which letters are for and which against the graffiti artist?

b Which letter was written by one of the speakers in Task 1? Give reasons for your choice.

c Write a letter to the newspaper expressing your point of view.

- How can you say such a thing?
- Oh, come on.
- I disagree.
- I'm afraid I just can't understand your attitude.

LEARNING STRATEGY

Cooperating = sharing ideas with other students and learning together.

Task 3

a Pair Work Decide what you think should happen to Dennis Wilson. Take opposing sides. Use the expressions in the model at left.

b Pair Work Change partners and roles and do the task again.

Task 4

a Group Work Discussion. What would you do if you saw some people spraying graffiti on a wall? Make a list of options.

b Group Work Compare options with another group.

Language Focus 2 Idioms

1 a Look at the following idioms (in italics) and match them with their meanings.

Idioms

1 My friends enjoyed the speeches at the political rally, but I thought that they were *a lot of hot air*.
2 I'm *having second thoughts* about going out with Lucio because he never has any money.
3 Ron really *put his foot in his mouth* when he let on about the surprise party for Nick.
4 Naomi's really been *throwing her weight around* since she got that promotion.
5 Renata's been so down since her boyfriend left that I finally had to tell her to *snap out of it*.
6 My brother *hit it off* so well with his new girlfriend that they decided to get married after dating for only a month.
7 I had to *bite my tongue* when the boss started telling those tasteless jokes.
8 After listening to the front office staff gossiping about everyone else in the office, I finally had to *give them a piece of my mind*.

Meaning

.... to consider changing one's mind
.... to speak severely to someone over whom you have authority
.... to say something extremely indiscrete
.... to speak a lot, but in a way that makes very little sense
.... to use one's authority
.... to make an effort to overcome negative feelings
.... to get along well with someone on first meeting them
.... to keep silent when you really want to speak

"Ron really said something stupid when he let on about the surprise party for Nick."

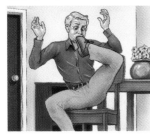

b Now rewrite the statements using the example on the left.

c PairWork Compare statements with another student.

2 a PairWork Match the following questions/statements and responses and practice them.

Questions/Statements

1 How was your date?
2 What did you think when you heard the news?
3 I've decided to marry Mickey.
4 When do you want to get together?
5 What did you do when he asked for help?

Responses

.... You must be out of your mind.
.... I bent over backwards, but it didn't make any difference.
.... I don't know. Just get in touch.
.... I couldn't believe my ears.
.... He turned out to be a real pain in the neck.

b PairWork Take turns making statements or asking questions. Use the above responses to your partner's statements or questions.

Language Focus 2: Idioms

1 (a) In this task students use the situation or context to make intelligent guesses about the meanings of each idiom. Have students read each sentence silently, at least twice. Read aloud to the whole class the list of meanings. Then have students make their choices. Elicit answers from around the class.
(Answers: 1—to speak a lot, but in a way that makes very little sense; 2—to consider changing one's mind; 3—to say something extremely indiscrete; 4—to use one's authority; 5—to make an effort to overcome negative feelings; 6—to get along well with someone on first meeting them; 7—to keep silent when you really want to speak; 8—to speak severely to)

(b) This is an individual writing task. Students rephrase the statements, using the meanings rather than the idioms, and following the example of the sample language. They will need to change the pronouns to match those in the original sentence. Circulate and correct spelling and grammar.

(c) In pairs, students read each other's work and discuss any differences of opinion about the grammar.

2. (a) In pairs, students match each statement/question with the right response. Then have the students in each pair practice asking and answering (or stating and responding). Make sure that students switch roles after they have completed the list.
(Answers: 1—He turned out to be a real pain in the neck. 2—I couldn't believe my ears. 3—You must be out of your mind. 4—I don't know. Just get in touch. 5—I bent over backwards, but it didn't make any difference.)

(b) Before the pair activity, have each student think of at least one question or statement for each of the responses in the book. Do one example first with the whole class. Circulate and provide help if necessary as students ask their questions and their partners answer by using the appropriate response from the list.

Self-Check

Communication Challenge

Challenge 14 is on pages 125 and 127 of the student text, and suggestions for its use are on page 125 in this Teacher's Extended Edition.

1. Encourage students to complete this task without looking back at the unit.

2. Students think about when and where they might talk about cultural attitudes and beliefs or express a point of view. Ask them to be as specific as possible. Encourage them to think about situations they have been in when they needed to use this language. **Optional.** In class, students compare their responses with others. Elicit responses from around the class.

3. Students will probably need to bring in photographs or drawings of the street art that they find. Lead the class in a discussion about the general and relative merits of street art. Make sure that students support their opinions on this issue.

4. Have students work individually to check off the words that they know.

• The grammar summary for this unit is on page 134.

Self-Check

COMMUNICATION CHALLENGE
Group Work Work in two groups. Group A: Look at Challenge 14A on page 125. Group B: Look at Challenge 14B on page 127.

1 Write three new sentences or questions you learned.

....

....

....

2 Review the language skills you practiced in this unit. In what situations might you use this language?

WHEN WOULD YOU USE THIS LANGUAGE?

	Situations
Talk about cultural attitudes and beliefs	
Express a point of view	

3 Out of Class Find examples of graffiti, slogans, etc. in your neighborhood. Bring them to class and be prepared to discuss them in English. Alternative: If possible, bring photographs of "street art" to class and discuss them. Do they have any value or not?

	DOES IT HAVE VALUE?	
EXAMPLE OF GRAFFITI	**YES**	**NO**

4 Vocabulary check. Check [√] the words you know.

Adjectives/Adverbs

☐ aboriginal	☐ destructive	☐ sarcastic
☐ academic	☐ fake	☐ serious
☐ artificial	☐ high-spirited	☐ sophisticated
☐ certain	☐ lightly	☐ temporary
☐ clever	☐ magical	☐ terminal
☐ considered	☐ religious	☐ unlucky

Nouns

☐ credibility	☐ mural	☐ spray can
☐ euphemism	☐ options	☐ supernatural
☐ graffiti	☐ origins	☐ taboo
magic	☐ popularity	☐ vandal
☐ marketer	☐ sale	

Verbs

☐ cancel	☐ express	☐ turn off
☐ check	☐ mention	☐ uphold
☐ cooperate	☐ prohibit	
☐ cure	☐ punish	

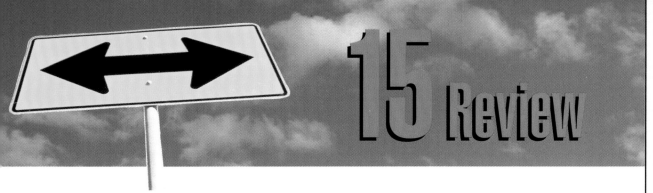

15 Review

Task 1

Pretend that you are one of these people. Make up a story surrounding the pictures. Think about these questions and make notes.

1 Where did it take place?
2 Who were your companions?
3 What was the most frightening thing about the whole incident?
4 How did your companions react?
5 What did you expect was going to happen?
6 What happened immediately after the incident pictured happened?
7 What did you suggest doing?
8 What were you supposed to have done that would have prevented the incident?

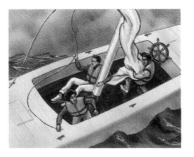 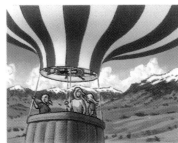 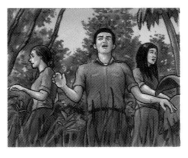

Task 2

a Classify these words.

suggest   intend   remind   want   ask
consider demand   expect   hope deny

WORDS TO DESCRIBE MENTAL STATES	WORDS TO REPORT WHAT SOMEONE SAYS

Task 1.   Recounting stories or events is an important discourse skill. Students choose one of the pictures to create a story about. They imagine they are the person in the picture and use the questions provided as a guide. Have them make notes rather than writing the story out in full. **Variation.** Ask students to choose one of the pictures and create their story for it outside class, before the lesson. Then they retell their story in small groups, referring to their notes as little as possible. If the listeners need anything in the story clarified or explained, they should ask questions. Circulate and monitor content and pronunciation.

Task 2.   (a) Remind students that grouping words is one important way of learning new vocabulary and that they can group words in many different ways—for example, words that mean the same or similar things, words that look similar, or words about the same topic or subject. Then have students fill out the chart. (Answers: Words to Describe Mental States—consider, intend, expect, want, hope; Words to Report What Someone Says—suggest, demand, remind, ask, deny)

(b) Do this as an individual reading task. Students read the sentences and then fill in the blanks with the appropriate words. Elicit responses from around the class.
(Answers: 1—consider; 2—suggest; 3—intend; 4—ask; 5—want)

(c) In pairs, students develop three questions, using the words from the list, and practice asking and answering them. Circulate and monitor content and pronunciation. Elicit answers from around the class.

Communication Challenge

Challenge 15 is on pages 120, 123, and 128 of the student text, and suggestions for its use are on page 120 in this Teacher's Extended Edition.

Task 3. **(a, b)** 🎧 This task practices selective listening. Play the tape and have students listen to the responses. Have them make a note of each person's response. Then play the tape again so that students can infer what questions had prompted the responses. Have students fill out the chart.
(Suggested answers: What is your favorite activity? Di—walking along the beach; Steve—lying down and listening to music. What would you most like to do? Di—climb Mt. Everest without oxygen; Steve—learn to paint. What's the hardest thing you ever did? Di—having a baby in the bathroom; Steve—finishing his college degree. What's the worst thing that ever happened to you? Di—getting caught criticizing some friends' daughter; Steve—having his leg broken in a car accident. What's the best thing that ever happened to you? Di—having the baby; Steve—getting to meet Bob Dylan after an anniversary concert)

(c) In groups, students take turns asking the questions. One person in the group records, in note form only, the answers that group members give. Call on groups to report their answers to the whole class.

COMMUNICATION CHALLENGE

Group Work Student A: Look at Challenge 15A on page 120. Student B: Look at Challenge 15B on page 123. Student C: Look at Challenge 15C on page 128.

b Fill in the blanks with the most appropriate word from the chart.

1 What languages other than English would you .... learning if you had the choice?
2 What do you .... we do after class?
3 What do you .... to do during the next vacation?
4 What would you most like to .... the teacher about his/her personal life?
5 As a child, what did you most .... to be when you grew up?
6 _____ ?
7 _____ ?
8 _____ ?

c **Pair Work** Add three questions of your own using words from the list, and take turns asking and answering questions.

Task 3

a 🎧 Listen. You will hear two people answering five questions. Make a note of their responses.

	Questions	Di	Steve
1			
	?		
2			
	?		
3			
	?		
4			
	?		
5			
	?		

b **Pair Work** Study the responses and guess what the questions were. Write the questions in the blank lines above.

c **Group Work** Take turns asking each other these questions. One person records the answers and reports them to the class.

Communication Challenges

Challenge 1

a **Pair Work** Imagine that your school is 100 years old this year. Plan a week-long festival to celebrate the event. Decide when it will be held, who will be invited, what events will be staged. Now write a program.

b **Group Work** Work with another pair and ask them about their festival program.

c **Group Work** Put the programs on the classroom walls. Circulate and decide which group has the best program.

d Take turns telling the rest of the class about your festival and inviting them to come.

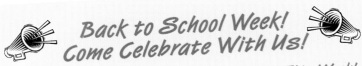

Back to School Week! Come Celebrate With Us!

Atlas School is One Hundred Years Old This Week!

 MONDAY
Evening Celebration Concert: Hear the Atlas School Symphony Orchestra conducted by Akron Symphony Orchestra's Maestro Steven Challenor, one of our most famous graduates.

 TUESDAY
Gala Track Meet: Show your prowess in track and field events at this very special all-day sporting carnival. Meet Gloria Day, 200 meter Olympic sprint champion.

 WEDNESDAY
Honor our oldest alumni at a special afternoon tea ceremony. The guest of honor will be celebrated 95-year-old author Jack Richards.

 THURSDAY
On Thursday evening, join the Board of Governors and distinguished guests at the opening of the new Access Learning Center.

 FRIDAY
Quiz Night! Get a group of friends together and test your general knowledge. There will be great prizes for the winning teams.

SATURDAY/SUNDAY
All the fun of the fair! Help the week go out with a bang with two days of fun, music, competitions, and prizes at the Grand Finale Fair.

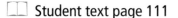

Communication Challenge 1

The Communication Challenge tasks provide opportunities for students to use, in a freer context, the language they have been learning.

With the whole class, first discuss the different language tasks that are included here. Students will need to use their knowledge and experience as well as their imagination to come up with ideas for a celebration. They negotiate these ideas with a partner, agree on a final plan of events, and then write their plan as a program so that others can follow it. The program should be written large enough to be used as a wall poster. Students can use the example here as a model if they wish.

(a) In this first phase, make sure that students are as specific as possible. Circulate and provide help when necessary.

(b) Combine two pairs and have them compare and discuss their programs.

(c) Each pair puts its program up, and the students wander around the room reading each one.

(d) Make this a role-playing activity. Encourage students to "sell" their program by describing it in the most positive way.

Communication Challenge 2A, 2B, and 2C

Challenge 2A is on this page, Challenge 2B is on page 114, and Challenge 2C is on page 116. Divide the class into three groups, one to take the role of Student A, one Student B, and one Student C.

Task 1

• Student A: (a) Have students read the information silently, and then provide clarification if needed.
(b) Have students work in their groups to determine the specific questions they will ask. Circulate and monitor the interviews. Make sure that students refer as little as possible to notes and ask or answer from memory.

Task 2.
Reorganize the groups so that each interviewer tells his or her story of the rescue to a new group.

• Student B: These students read the information and take notes. They then try to memorize the information so that they can answer without having to consult their notes.

• Student C: These students read the information and take notes. They then try to memorize the information so they can answer without having to consult their notes.

Communication Challenge 3

(a) Have pairs of students choose the country they will move to and even the region or city. Then they brainstorm ideas for meeting people and finding out about the country. Encourage them to think about their own experiences when they compile their list.
(b) Combine two pairs so that students work in small groups. From the ideas that students have already discussed in their pairs, have them compile a list of ten. They then negotiate which ideas are most/least interesting and most/least practical, and rank them in order.
(c) With the whole class, compare ideas and have the class vote on the most interesting list. **Variation.** Have the class vote on the most practical list.

Challenge 2A

Task 1

Student A

a You are a journalist. You are interviewing two people together, one who was lost for several days on a remote island and the person who found him/her. You are going to write a story about the incident, and need to know the following information:

- how he/she got lost
- how he/she felt while he/she was lost
- what he/she ate and drank
- how long he/she was lost
- what things happened to him/her
- how he/she was found
- how he/she felt when he/she was found

b Interview the person who was lost, and then the person who found him/her. Ask questions and make a note of similarities and differences in the facts and opinions of the two people.

Task 2

Now use your notes to tell the story to another group.

Challenge 3

A I'd take classes in ceramics.

B I had no idea you were interested in ceramics.

A I'm not, but it's such a boring hobby, there must be lots of interesting conversations in the class.

B That's a crazy idea. I'd find out about the place before I go. I'd check the encyclopedia and I'd visit the local consulate. They always have lots of information.

a **Pair Work** You've just moved, or are about to move, to another country to start a position as a computer programmer with a large company. You know very little about this country. Brainstorm ideas for meeting people and finding out about your new country.

b **Group Work** Work with another pair, and write down ten ideas. Rank the ideas from most to least interesting (1 = most interesting). Now rank them again from most to least practical (1 = most practical).

IDEAS	INTERESTING	PRACTICAL
1		
2		
3		
4		
5		
6		
7		
8		
9		
10		

c **Group Work** Compare lists. Which pair has the most interesting ideas overall?

Challenge 4

a 🎧 Listen to four people talking about someone they live with and make a list of the individuals' positive and negative points.

b **Pair Work** Decide which of the people you would like to live with and which you would not like to live with.

Challenge 6A

"I asked if they could put the CDs back in their cases and then put them on the bookshelf."

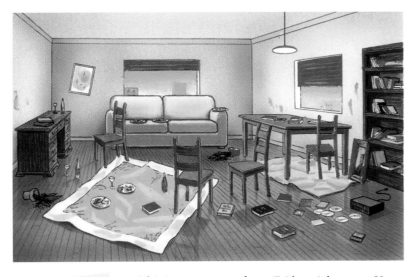

CDs back in cases on bookshelf
bottles and glasses in garbage bags
plates in garbage bags
marks cleaned off wall
rugs straightened out
books back in bookcase
paintings hung back on wall
potted plant picked up and put on balcony
chairs put around table
CD player plugged in and put on desk

This is your room after a Friday night party. Your roommate is returning from a vacation the following day. Some of your friends say that they will stay and clean up because you're going away for the weekend, and you want the room fixed before your roommate returns. You give them a note with the following instructions. Call your roommate and ask if your instructions were carried out. Tell him/her what you wanted done.

Communication Challenge 4

(a) 🎧 This is a selective listening task. Play the tape as many times as is necessary, and allow students to take notes.

(b) In pairs, students compare their responses and express their judgments about which of the four people they would most like to have as a roommate and which one they would least like. Make sure that they give reasons for their preferences.

Communication Challenge 6A and 6B

Challenge 6A is on this page. Challenge 6B is on page 116. Divide the class into two groups, one to take the role of Student A and one to take the role of Student B.

• Have students who are playing the role of Student A study the list of chores and try to memorize it. They will "call" their roommate (Student B) and describe what they wanted done and ask whether their friends have indeed completed all the tasks. As much as possible, students should avoid referring to the list during the phone call.

• Students who are playing the role of Student B should examine the illustration of the cleaned-up room and, using the sample language as a model, respond to Student A's queries.

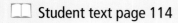
Communication Challenge 2B

See page 112 for suggestions for using Challenge 2A, 2B, and 2C.

Challenge 2B

Student B

You have just been rescued from a remote island, and are talking to a journalist who wants to know what happened. Also present is the person who rescued you.

You were flying your light plane off the coast when the engine failed. You managed to land on the beach of an uninhabited island. Amazingly, you were not hurt. Think about how you felt when the accident happened, and what you ate and drank. You walked into the center of the island and slept in a cave. You were there for about a week. One night, you had a dream in which a friend told you to walk back to the coast. You did so, and when you got there you saw a boat. You lit a fire, and the person on the boat saw the fire and rescued you. Think about how you felt when you were rescued.

Key to Warm-up Quiz (page 51)
(Answers are in boldface.)

Question 1: The dodo is **(a) an extinct animal** (b) a make believe creature
(c) a living animal
Question 2: The giant panda is an endangered animal. **True** or false.
Question 3: Kangaroos are considered gourmet food in Australia. True or **false.**
Question 4: Elephants are used as working animals in **(a) Thailand** (b) Singapore
(c) Taiwan.
Question 5: Kiwis are (a) small horses **(b) birds** (c) make believe creatures
Question 6: Elderly people who have pets tend to live longer than those who live alone.
True or false?

Challenge 7A

Task 1

a You want to go on an eco-tourism trip, so you picked up a couple of brochures. Now you have to decide which of these trips would be best to take. You go to see a travel agent who has more information about each trip.

b Ask the travel agent questions to find out which trip . . .
- is the most exciting.
- is the most dangerous.
- lets you see the most exotic animals.
- lets you see the most endangered species.
- takes you to the most mysterious places.
- has the most extreme weather.
- is the most unusual.
- is the cheapest.

c Ask any other questions you like and decide which trip you are going to take, and why.

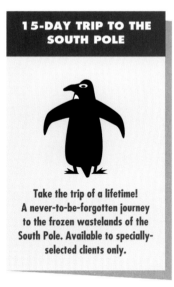

15-DAY TRIP TO THE SOUTH POLE

Take the trip of a lifetime! A never-to-be-forgotten journey to the frozen wastelands of the South Pole. Available to specially-selected clients only.

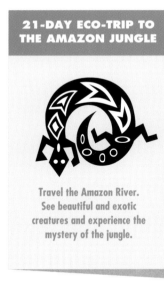

21-DAY ECO-TRIP TO THE AMAZON JUNGLE

Travel the Amazon River. See beautiful and exotic creatures and experience the mystery of the jungle.

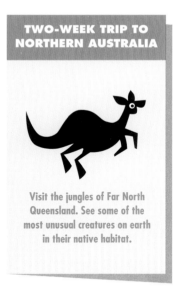

TWO-WEEK TRIP TO NORTHERN AUSTRALIA

Visit the jungles of Far North Queensland. See some of the most unusual creatures on earth in their native habitat.

Task 2

Now change roles and do the task again.

Communication Challenge 7A and 7B

Challenge 7A is on this page. Challenge 7B is on page 117. Divide the class into two groups, one to take the role of the tourist and the other to take the role of the travel agent.

- The first group examines the brochures to get a sense of what vacation they might like. Then they ask whether a particular trip is exciting, dangerous, etc., until they have covered all the items on the list. Then this group asks new questions of their own making, discusses the travel agent's responses, and votes on which trip to take.

- The second group examines the "additional information" and provides the first group with answers to their questions. Then students switch roles and go through the process again.

Communication Challenge 2C

See page 112 for suggestions for using Challenge 2A, 2B, and 2C.

Communication Challenge 6B

See page 113 for suggestions for using Challenge 6A and 6B.

Challenge 2C

Student C

You are taking part in an interview between a journalist and a person you rescued from an island. You were on a sailing trip when you saw the wreckage of a light plane in the water. You had heard on the news that the plane had been missing for four days. You went ashore and found the person who looked frightened and confused. He/She had had nothing to eat or drink and had not slept while on the island.

Challenge 6B

"Well, the CDs have been put back in their cases, but they've been put on the desk, not on the bookcase."

You've just returned from a vacation and you receive a call from your roommate who had a party while you were away. He/She asked his/her friends to clean up after the party because he/she had to go away for the weekend. Listen to what the friends were asked to do and then say what they really did.

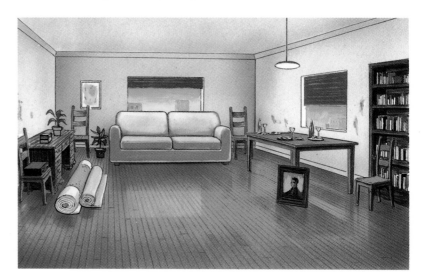

Challenge 7B

Task 1

You are a travel agent. A customer comes in with several brochures. You look up the following additional information to help him/her decide which trip to take. Be prepared to answer other questions as well.

Task 2

Now change roles and do the task again.

15-DAY TRIP TO THE SOUTH POLE

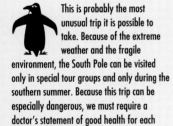

This is probably the most unusual trip it is possible to take. Because of the extreme weather and the fragile environment, the South Pole can be visited only in special tour groups and only during the southern summer. Because this trip can be especially dangerous, we must require a doctor's statement of good health for each client. It isn't cheap, but it's unique.

21-DAY ECO-TRIP TO THE AMAZON JUNGLE

This boat trip is probably the most exciting one we offer. Clients travel to the mysterious upper reaches of the Amazon River, where they see the most exotic wildlife on earth. Travel in the jungle can be dangerous, although we haven't lost a client yet! The trip is reasonably priced.

TWO-WEEK TRIP TO NORTHERN AUSTRALIA

This trip is a must for clients who are interested in wildlife. They will have a chance to see many unusual and endangered species including the extremely rare Northern Tree Kangaroo. The great distances make this one of the more expensive trips we offer.

Challenge 8A

* image of company should be dignified
* wants to appeal to people with good taste
* doesn't want to spend too much on the advertising campaign
* need to develop a product range that can be worn in both casual and formal situations

Task 1

Student A

Work with Students B and C to design a corporate image, including a logo and slogan for a clothing company. Use the following notes which you made while interviewing the Managing Director.

Task 2

Student B

When you have finished, compare your logo and slogan with another group.

Communication Challenge 7B

See page 115 for suggestions for using Challenge 7A and 7B.

Communication Challenge 8A, 8B, and 8C

Challenge 8A is on this page, Challenge 8B is on page 118, and Challenge 8C is on page 120. Divide the class into three groups, one to take the role of Student A, one Student B, and one Student C.

• Each group of students consists of one Student A, one Student B, and one Student C. Each student has been given a different set of information. Together, they design a corporate logo and slogan. Then the groups compare their products with other groups.

Communication Challenge 8B

See page 116 for suggestions for using Challenge 8A, 8B, and 8C.

Communication Challenge 9

Task 1. (a) Have students work in groups of at least four. They choose a cause from the list and decide how they could raise money for the cause and what other types of help would benefit the cause.

(b) Groups discuss those aspects of the cause that are most attractive and appealing. Explain that for the group presentation, students may choose different communication modes to persuade others to support their cause. For example, they may want to write or draw something for others to read while they are speaking to the class. Set a time limit of five minutes for the presentation.

Task 2. (a) With the whole class, decide on a framework for judging each presentation and the cause it recommends. Have those students watching the presentation make notes on what is presented as well as how it is presented. Have them consider information, interest, and clarity.

(b) Have students vote on which cause to support.

Challenge 8B

Task 1

Student B

Work with Students A and C to design a corporate image, including a logo and slogan for a clothing company. Use the following notes which you made while interviewing the Personnel Manager.

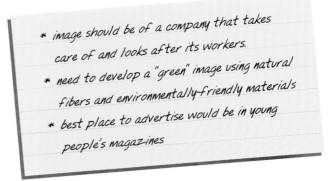

* image should be of a company that takes care of and looks after its workers.
* need to develop a "green" image using natural fibers and environmentally-friendly materials
* best place to advertise would be in young people's magazines

Task 2

Compare your logo and slogan with another group.

Challenge 9

Task 1

a **Group Work** Look again at the various tasks in Chain 1 on pages 68–69. Each group should select a different cause and prepare a plan to support it. Decide how to raise money and think about other kinds of volunteer support that you might get.

b **Group Work** Decide what you would say to get the different kinds of support. Prepare a group presentation.

Task 2

a **Group Work** Class presentation. Take turns presenting your cause to the rest of the class.

b **Group Work** Now vote on which cause to support.

Challenge 11A

Task 1

With the information you have available, decide which of these people would be the best to . . .

- work with ....
- prepare for an exam with ....
- hang out with ....
- have around in an emergency ....

NAME	AT WORK	AT HOME	AT PLAY
Maurice	always in a hurry to get things done; gets upset when things go wrong	?	loves to play sports and competitive games; gets upset when he loses
Kim	?	doesn't mind a messy place as long as it's clean	?
Jodie	doesn't mind when things go wrong; is the first to take a coffee break	?	great conversationalist; enjoys physical team sports but is not very good at board games
Kerry	?	likes to organize others	?

Task 2

a Ask your partner questions about the behavior of these people and complete the missing parts of the chart.

b Now work with your partner to decide who would be the best person . . .

- to work with ....
- to prepare for an exam with ....
- to hang out with ....
- to have around in an emergency ....

Communication Challenge 11A and 11B

Challenge 11A is on this page. Challenge 11B is on page 121. Divide the class into two groups, one to work with the information in 11A and the other to work with the information in 11B. Have students work in pairs, with each pair made up of one working on 11A and the other working on 11B.

Task 1. Each student decides which of the four people would be the best choice in terms of the four categories.

Task 2. (a) Each student then asks his or her partner for the missing information.

(b) Together, they work to determine which of the four people would be the best choice in light of the completed chart.

Communication Challenge 8C

See page 116 for suggestions for using Challenge 8A, 8B, and 8C.

Communication Challenge 15A, 15B, and 15C

Challenge 15A is on this page, Challenge 15B is on page 123, and Challenge 15C is on page 128. Divide the class into three groups, one to read Susan's story, one to read George's story, and one to read Yvonne's story.

• After each group of students has read the assigned story, have them come together, discuss what they have read, and try to establish which of the three figures is the most pessimistic. Make sure that students can back up their opinions.

Challenge 8C

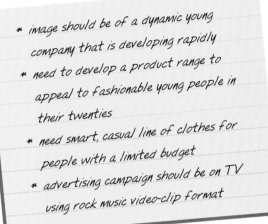

* image should be of a dynamic young company that is developing rapidly
* need to develop a product range to appeal to fashionable young people in their twenties
* need smart, casual line of clothes for people with a limited budget
* advertising campaign should be on TV using rock music video-clip format

Task 1

Student C

Work with Students A and B to design a corporate image, including a logo and slogan for a clothing company. Use the following notes which you made while interviewing the Advertising Manager.

Task 2

When you have finished, compare your logo and slogan with another group.

Challenge 15A

Who is the most optimistic? Who is the most pessimistic? Report to your partners what Susan says, and decide.

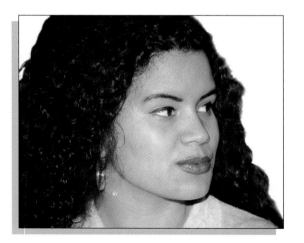

❝I think that childhood was the best time in my life, so I guess in some ways I'm a little more backward-looking than many people. On the other hand, I don't believe that the environment has deteriorated as much as the media suggests. I don't think that I'll be better off as I get older, either. And I don't think I'm as well off as my parents were at my age. ❞

Challenge 11B

Task 1

With the information you have available, decide which of these people would be the best person to . . .

- work with   ....
- prepare for an exam with   ....
- hang out with   ....
- have around in an emergency   ....

NAME	AT WORK	AT HOME	AT PLAY
Maurice	?	often takes work home so has little time for family and friends	?
Kim	often arrives late for work; enjoys the routine of work but does not like new challenges	?	is good at introducing people to each other; a good mixer and sympathetic listener
Jodie	?	likes to take frequent vacations so is not often at home	?
Kerry	is constantly applying for new jobs; usually tries to do several things at once	?	talks about self a lot but is amusing company at parties; likes to win at games

Task 2

a Ask your partner questions about the behavior of these people and complete the missing parts of the chart.

b Now work with your partner to decide who would be the best person . . .

- to work with   ....
- to prepare for an exam with   ....
- to hang out with   ....
- to have around in an emergency   ....

Communication Challenge 11B

See page 119 for suggestions for using Challenge 11A and 11B.

Communication Challenge 12A and 12B

Challenge 12A is on this page. Challenge 12B is on page 124. Divide the class into two groups, one to play the role of Student A and the other to play the role of Student B. Have students work in pairs, with each pair made up of one student working on 12A and the other working on 12B.

Task 1. Each student first considers the information provided to him or her. Then the partners share information so that they can make notes about the four people and then come to agreement about which one should be their leader.

Task 2. Combine pairs and have them compare their choices and discuss the reasoning they used to make their respective choices.

Challenge 12A

Task 1

Student A

You are trapped in a remote place with the following people. Here is what other people said about them. Which one will you elect as your leader? Work with Student B to make notes on each person and then decide.

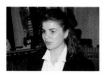

Graciela's boss: "I don't have too many complaints about Graciela. She's independent—in fact she's a bit of a loner. She also tends not to listen to others."

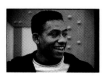

Conrad's coworker: "The good thing about working with Conrad is that he gets things done. He's really self-motivated."

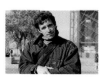

Steve's housemate: "I used to share an apartment with Steve, but I moved out because he was always criticizing the others in the apartment. Also, he'd get angry if we had to decide on something, and the decision didn't go his way—you know, he's one of those guys who always has to get his own way."

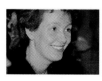

Rebecca's teacher: "Rebecca was one of my favorite students. She is a very persistent person—never gives up. She was also very good at getting others involved in things."

	POSITIVE	NEGATIVE
Graciela		
Conrad		
Stephen		
Rebecca		

Task 2

Now compare your choice with another pair.

Challenge 15B

Who is the most optimistic? Who is the most pessimistic? Report to your partners what George says, and decide.

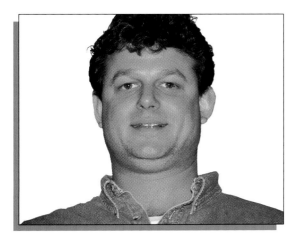

" I have a good life, and I expect to be better off as I get older. I'm certainly better off financially than I was when I was in my twenties. On the other hand, I don't think that my children will be as well off as I am. I think that there will be fewer educational and employment opportunities and with all the environmental problems we are facing, I don't think that the world will be as pleasant a place to live. Unfortunately, science doesn't seem to be able to provide solutions to major problems such as AIDS, and environmental problems. "

📖 Student text page 123

Communication Challenge 15B

See page 120 for suggestions for using Challenge 15A, 15B, and 15C.

Communication Challenge 12B

See page 122 for suggestions for using Challenge 12A and 12B.

Task 1

Student B

You are trapped in a remote place with the following people. Here is what other people said about them. Which one will you elect as your leader? Work with Student A to make notes on each person and then decide.

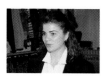

Graciela's coworker: "I don't mind working with her at all. Graciela has a very strong personality, which might put some people off, but I think it's a positive thing. She's also good at communicating her ideas."

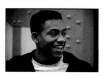

Conrad's boss: "I had to move Conrad to another part of the firm. He wasn't good at getting others to do things, and would tend to do them himself rather than getting the cooperation of the people he was working with."

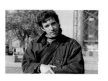

Steve's teacher: "I always knew that Steve would become an artist or a designer. In school, he always had very creative ideas, and came up with interesting solutions to problems."

Rebecca's ex-boyfriend: "I guess we split up because our personalities are so different. I'm easygoing, very laid back. Rebecca's the driven type. She was always getting impatient when people didn't understand what she was talking about."

	POSITIVE	NEGATIVE
Graciela		
Conrad		
Stephen		
Rebecca		

Task 2

Now compare your choice with another pair.

Challenge 14 A

Task 1

Brainstorm. Think of up to five arguments *in favor of* the following statement: "Young people who paint graffiti on other people's property are destructive vandals who ought to be punished."

1 ....

2 ....

3 ....

4 ....

5 ....

Task 2

a Select three or four people to speak against the following statement: "Young people who paint graffiti on other people's property are destructive vandals who ought to be punished."

b The speakers take ten minutes to prepare their arguments and decide who is to say what.

c The rest of the group make a checklist of points for and against the statement.

Task 3

a Each speaker has three minutes to state his/her case. Alternate between those speaking for and against.

b As they speak, the rest of the class uses the checklist developed in Task 2 to evaluate which points have been covered.

Task 4

The class votes on which side presented the best case.

Communication Challenge 14A and 14B

Challenge 14A is on this page, and Challenge 14B is on page 127. Have the whole class complete Challenge 14A before moving to Challenge 14B.

Task 1. Guide the brainstorming by encouraging students to first consider arguments in favor of the statement. Explain to the class that arguing in favor means using extra information to support the original idea/statement. People might support their main idea or opinion by giving extra information—for example, statistics—or by giving examples from their own or other people's personal experience.

Task 2. (a) Three or four students argue against the statement. If possible, choose volunteers.
(b) Give them time together to discuss what they will say.
(c) As the speakers prepare their arguments, the rest of the class works in a group to make their own checklist on arguments both for and against.

Task 3. (a) Limit the speaking to three minutes, with the first speaker "for" followed by a speaker "against," and continue this pattern.
(b) As each speaker talks to the class, have the listeners make notes on the arguments the speaker gives and compare these with their checklist.

Task 4. The whole class votes on the best argument.

Communication Challenge 13

Task 1. Have students complete this task in small groups.
(Answers, top to bottom: 4, 7, 12, 10, 9, 14, 8, 5, 3, 1, 6, 2, 11, 13)

Task 2. Each group makes up an ending for the story. This can be a writing task, with one member of the group taking dictation. Swap papers and have groups read each other's endings. If you use this as an oral exercise, have one member of the group retell the whole story to the class after the group has written its new ending.

Challenge 13

Task 1

Study the following events and put them in order (1 to 14).

.... While Jack was in the store, his car was towed away.

.... When he got to her house, he found that he didn't have enough money to pay for the taxi.

.... She said that she'd never forget her birthday.

.... She'd been waiting over two hours when he finally arrived.

.... He was supposed to have arrived at seven, but didn't get there till after 9:30.

.... She said that she didn't believe him, because she'd called his office and no one had answered.

.... Jack had to ask his girlfriend for a loan.

.... He tried to take a bus, but they were all full.

.... He parked in a no parking zone.

.... Jack decided to drive to his girlfriend's place to take her out for her birthday.

.... In the end, he had to take a taxi.

.... He stopped on the way to buy her some flowers.

.... She was very angry and upset.

.... He lied and said that he'd been delayed at work by the boss, because he was embarrassed about the car being towed.

Task 2

Make up an ending to the story and tell it to another group.

Challenge 14B

Task 1

Brainstorm. Think of up to five arguments *in favor of* the following statement: "Young people who paint murals on public property are creative artists who ought to be rewarded."

1 ....

2 ....

3 ....

4 ....

5 ....

Task 2

a Select three or four people to speak against the following statement: "Young people who paint murals on public property are creative artists who ought to be rewarded."

b The speakers take ten minutes to prepare their arguments and decide who is to say what.

c The rest of the group make a checklist of points for and against the statement.

Task 3

a Each speaker has three minutes to state his/her case. Alternate between those speaking for and against.

b As they speak, the rest of the class uses the checklist developed in Task 2 to evaluate which points have been covered.

Task 4

The class votes on which side presented the best case.

📖 Student text page 127

Communication Challenge 14B

See page 125 for suggestions for using Challenge 14A and 14B.

Communication Challenge 15C

See page 120 for suggestions for using Challenge 15A, 15B, and 15C.

Challenge 15C

Who is the most optimistic? Who is the most pessimistic? Report to your partners what Yvonne says, and decide.

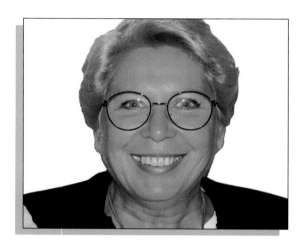

" I'll be fifty-five next birthday, and so I've seen a lot of changes taking place. I've seen the world come to the brink of nuclear war. I've seen footage of famine in Africa. But for me, life keeps getting better and better. I'm certainly a lot better off than I was when I was young, and I'm better off than my parents were when they were in their fifties. I think that science has the potential to solve the problems we face. **"**

Grammar Summaries

Unit 1

1 Prepositional phrases

We lived *on the floor* above the noisiest people on the block.
It was pointless trying to sleep *during the festival*.
We waited *for hours* but he never came back.
They went *into the bus station* when the storm started.
They waited *in the bus station* until the storm passed.
Holding the party *on a boat* was a stroke of genius.
Getting *into the program* was a real challenge.
Unfortunately, the joke went *over their heads*.
I haven't been back there *since they threw me out*.
We went *to the jazz festival* together last year.
They came *towards us* looking threatening.
I walked *under the ladder* to show I wasn't superstitious.
I trained *until eight o'clock*.

2 Modals: *can/could/would/would mind*

Can you make it to the party?	Yes, I can.	No, I can't.
Could you invite Mike as well?	Yes, I could.	No, I couldn't.
Would you be able to come at around eight?	Yes, I would.	No, I wouldn't.
Would they mind if I brought a friend?	Yes, they would.	No, they wouldn't.

Unit 2

1 Short responses

A: Are you still reading that awful horoscope column in the newspaper?
B: Not since it said I'd win a million dollars.

A: Did you know that I saw a ghost once when I was a kid?
B: I find that hard to believe.

A: Have you seen the guy on TV who can bend spoons by looking at them?
B: No, not yet.

2 Relative adverbials: *where/when/why/how*

I don't really understand how it happened.
The place where it happened was about 50 kilometers from shore.
It was around 5 A.M. when I saw the lights of a tanker coming towards me.
The reason why they didn't see me was because of the huge waves.

Unit 3

1 Present perfect & simple past

Present perfect:

A state continuing from past to present
How long have you been here?
The store has been closed for hours.

Events in a time period leading up to the present
Have you seen the new movie at the Odeon?
I've decided I'm not the party type.

Past tense:

Habits or recurring events
Have you danced with him often?
I've been to ten parties in the last month.

Completed events at a definite time in the past
Did you go to the office party on Friday?
She didn't come to the party because she was sick.

2 Emphasis with *it* & *what*

What I love about my country is the political freedom.
It's the political freedom that I love about my country.
What annoys me about my job is having to work weekends.
It's having to work weekends that annoys me about my job.
What I admire about you is your patience.
It's your patience that I admire about you.

Unit 4

1 *When* & *if* clauses + modals *should/shouldn't*

What should I do if my co-workers smoke in the non-smoking areas at work?
If they smoke in the non-smoking areas, you shouldn't let them get away with it.
If they smoke in the non-smoking areas, you should ask them to stop.

What should I do when my brother comes in late and puts on loud music?
When he puts on loud music, you shouldn't just put up with it, you should ask him to turn it down.

2 Relative clauses with *whose/who/who is*

A: Would you like to share an apartment with someone who smokes?
B: I'd hate to share an apartment with someone who smokes.

A: Would you like to share a house with someone whose friends are always calling?
B: Sharing a house with someone whose friends are always calling wouldn't bother me at all, actually.

A: Would you like to live with someone who's extremely neat?
B: I couldn't stand living with someone who's extremely neat, because it would make me look like a slob.

Unit 6

1   Passives: past and perfect forms

A: When was that famous photo taken?
B: I think it was taken in the thirties. It's been around for many years.

A: Why was the exhibition cancelled?
B: There wasn't enough interest in the subject.

A: How were the pictures arranged?
B: They were put in chronological order—you know, by the year in which they were painted.

2   Reported speech

"Do you want these drinks?"   → She asked if we wanted those drinks.
"I put the book right here."   → He said that he had put the book right there.
"We wanted to meet you yesterday."   → Tony said that he had wanted to meet us the day before.

"I told you about the exam two days ago." → She said that she had told us about the exam two days earlier.

Unit 7

1   Relative clauses with *that* & *whose*

Reptiles are animals that have cold blood.
Reptiles are animals whose blood is cold.

Mammals are animals that have warm blood.
Mammals are animals whose blood is warm.

2   Superlative adjectives with present perfect

Who's the most interesting person you've ever met?   → Your brother, actually.
What's the most unusual thing you've ever done?   → Hang gliding in California.
What's the most frightening experience you've ever had? → Hang gliding in California.
Where's the most interesting place you've ever visited? → Oh, New York, without a doubt.
Why was the trip to Brazil so memorable?   → I made some fantastic friends.

Unit 8

1 Phrasal verbs + gerunds

Tracy's *looking forward to starting* the new job.
We'll have to *cut down on calling* your folks on the West Coast.
The boss decided not to *go through with firing* the front office guy.
Nina *put off telling* Jose she doesn't want to see him any more.
I intend to *keep on asking* her until she says "yes".
You should *cut down on going out* at night until after exams.
I'm not going to *put off telling* him what I think any longer.
They *plan on going* to Seoul for Chinese New Year.
I can't *put up with listening* to your complaints any longer.

2 Indirect questions & requests

Could you help us move the furniture?	→	I wonder if you could help us move the furniture.
Will it make a difference if we leave?	→	Do you think it will make a difference if we leave?
Does the new computer system get installed next week?	→	Can you tell me if the new computer system gets installed next week?
Could they borrow your car?	→	They wanted to know if they could borrow your car.
What is the teacher planning for us next week?	→	Can you tell me what the teacher is planning for us next week?

Unit 9

1 Object + infinitive

We want you to read the pamphlet carefully.
They'd like you to call them as soon as possible.
Tracy wants us to sign a petition on human rights.
I'd like you to get some information on Greenpeace for me.
Rebecca wants us to come over on Tuesday night.
Our class wants the whole school to contribute to the appeal.

2 Past conditional

If Winston hadn't become a volunteer aid worker, he wouldn't have gotten to Africa.
We'd never have raised the money if we hadn't all cooperated.
If my sister hadn't become a teacher, she would probably have become a social worker.
If the volunteer worker had been a bit more polite, I might have donated some money.
You wouldn't have gotten the job if you hadn't given that brilliant interview.
I'd have made an official complaint if it had been me who'd been fired.

Unit 11

1 *Wh-* questions + gerund/infinitive

How did you avoid going to the party last night?
What do you expect to do when you graduate?
Where do you hope to live when you return to Brazil?
Who would you consider asking to the party?
What do you intend to do over the weekend?
Why do you dislike watching sports on TV?
What kind of music do you enjoy listening to most?
Why did you deny going to the disco last night?
Why did she refuse to answer our questions?
Why do you want to go to the movies?
What did they suggest buying for the party?

2 Comparatives/superlative + gerund/infinitive

Growing up in the sixties was better than growing up in the seventies.
The best thing about being a child was not having to work.
Being an adult is much more interesting than being a child.
Living in a large city was more stressful than living in a small one.
Learning another language was the most difficult thing I've ever done.

Unit 12

1 Future perfect

I think that by the end of the century, the world population will have doubled.
Do you think that the economy will have improved by the end of the year?
This time next week, we'll have been here for over a year.
By tonight, I'll have spent over eight hours doing my assignment.
Paul thinks that by the end of the year he will have lost his job again.

2 Tag questions

They should have arrived by now, shouldn't they?
You weren't particularly interested in the position, were you?
Maria's been an organizer before, hasn't she?
We shouldn't spend too much time preparing for the interview, should we?
Most of the members of the class are hard-working, aren't they?
I wasn't that late, was I?

Unit 13

1 Review of past & perfect tenses

Simple past
Who lost their job last week?
Rick lost his job.
Susan didn't lose her job.

Present perfect
What's happened to you since we last met?
I've lost my job again.
They haven't found work since moving from the States.

Past perfect
Had you heard about the job before you read the ad?
I'd been in the job a week before anyone spoke to me.
We hadn't been there long before an argument broke out.

Present perfect progressive
Have you been waiting long?
I've been working for Langmore and Johns for three years.
We haven't been getting along lately.

Past progressive
Were you working for the Governor during his election campaign?
I was sitting at my desk when the boss came by and said he wanted to see me.
They weren't waiting for me when I stopped by to pick them up, so I drove on.

2 Supposed to have

A: Who was Adriana supposed to have called last night?
B: She was supposed to have called her parents, but she forgot.
A: What is something you are supposed to do by the end of the month?
B: I'm supposed to enroll for a computer course by Friday.

Unit 14

1 Complex passives

In many societies, it is considered bad taste to talk about money and wealth.
In other societies it is believed unlucky to talk about poverty.
Where I come from, it is thought impolite to ask how old someone is.
In years gone by, it was thought extremely rude to allow children to speak in front of adults.

2 Idioms

Tony thinks that most politicians are a lot of hot air.
I'm having second thoughts about buying a car since the cost of gas went up.
Tracy's really indiscrete—she's always putting her foot in her mouth.
I'm looking for another job because my boss is always throwing his weight around.
It doesn't help to be told to snap out of it when you're depressed about something.
Everyone in the new class is hitting it off so well that we decided to have a party.
I had to bite my tongue so I didn't insult your friend the other night when he was rude to me.
If the boss spoke to me like that, I'd give her a piece of my mind.

Credits

Photographs

Cover Sextant, Courtesy Peabody Essex Museum, Salem, MA. Photo by Mark Sexton; All maps Canada/ Rand McNally © Repolgle Globes; **9** © Superstock (c); © Randall Hyman/Stock Boston (bl) © Superstock (bc); © Keren Su/Stock Boston (br); © Jay Freis/The Image Bank (t); © Alan Becker/The Image Bank; (tl) **13** © Richard Pasley/Stock Boston; © Jonathan Stark/ Heinle & Heinle Publishers (all others); **15** © JS/H&H; **17** © JS/H&H (r, br, bl); © Hans Wendler/The Image Bank (t); Illustrations from The Rider-Waite® Tarot Deck reproduced by permission of U.S. Games Systems, Inc., Stamford, CT 06902 USA. Copyright © 1971 by U.S. Games Systems, Inc. Further reproduction prohibited. The Rider-Waite® Tarot Deck is a registered trademark of U.S. Games Systems, Inc. (tl); © Jay Freis/ The Image Bank; **20** © JS/H&H; **25** © Churchill & Klehr/Tony Stone Images, Inc. (l); © Dennis O'Clair/ Tony Stone Images, Inc. (r); © Claude Charlier/The Stock Market (bl); © David Nausbaum/ Tony Stone Images, Inc. (bcl); Catalyst/The Stock Market (bcr); © JS/H&H (br); Courtesy of Image Club/1-800-661-9410 (t); © Michael Melford/The Image Bank(tl); **26** © UPI/ Bettman; **28** © Superstock; **29** © JS/H&H (all); **31** © Stuart Cohen/Comstock **33** © JS/H&H (c, bl, bc, br);Courtesy of Image Club/1-800-661-9410 (t) **36** © JS/H&H; **39** © Bob Daemmrich/Stock Boston; **41** © JS/H&H (lc, ltc, lbc, lb); PhotoDisc ((t); © Garry Gay/The Image Bank (tl) **43** Joan Miró, *Head of a Catalan Peasant*, 1924–25. Oil. Courtesy of the Granger Collection. **44** © John Colletti/Stock Boston (t)); © JS/H&H (all others); **47** © JS/H&H (all); **51** © Superstock (l); © John Cancalosi/Stock Boston (c); © Comstock (bl); © JS/H&H (bcr); © Tom McCarthy/ PhotoEdit (br); © Don Klumpp/The Image Bank (t); © James Carmichael/The Image Bank (tl); **53** © Russ Kinne/ Photo Researchers; **55** © Comstock (tl); © Townsend P. Dickinson/Comstock (tr); © JS/H&H (bl); © Super- stock (br); **57** © Comstock; **59** © JS/H&H (all); © Frank Whitney/The Image Bank(t): **60** © JS/H&H; **62** © JS/H&H; **65** © JS/H&H; **67** © Anna E. Zuckerman/PhotoEdit (l); © Oxfam Hong Kong (r); © JS/H&H (bl); © Brent Jones/Stock Boston (br); Courtesy Project Bread, Boston, MA (t, tl); **68** Courtesy The French Library and Cultural Center, Inc., Boston, MA (cr); © JS/H&H (all others); **70** © Peter Erbland/ Aids Action Committee of Massachusetts, Inc.; **73** © Comstock; **75** © David Sailors/The Stock Market (l); © Superstock (r); © JS/H&H (bl); © Jon Feinghersh/ The Stock Market (br); PhotoDisc (t); © Garry Gay/ The Image Bank (tl) **77** © Comstock (r);

© JS/H&H (all others); © Pat Lacroix/The Image Bank (t); **78** © JS/H&H; **80** © JS/H&H; **81** © Linder Elem/ Stock Boston; **82** UPI/Bettman **83** © JS/H&H; **85** © Charles Gupton/The Stock Market(l); © Stacy Pickerell/Tony Stone Images, Inc. (r); © JS/H&H (bl); © Laura Elliott/Comstock (br); **86** © JS/H&H (all); **87** Lisa de George; **89** © Bob Daemmrich/Stock Boston; **93** © Jo Van Os/The Image Bank (t); © James H. Carmichael, Jr./The Image Bank **94** © The Granger Collection (l); © UPI/Bettman (c); © Bob Daemmrich/ Stock Boston (r); **98** © JS/H&H; **101** © Superstock (l); © JS/H&H (all others); © Gary S. Chapman/The Image Bank (t); © Lisa de George (tl); **105** © JS/H&H; **120** © JS/H&H; **122** © JS/H&H (all); **123** © JS/H&H; **124** © JS/H&H (all); **128** © JS/H&H

Illustrations

63 Lisa de George; **All others** Kevin Spaulding

Text

11 From Dragon Boat Festival brochure, courtesy of the Hong Kong Tourist Association. **19** From *Literary Outlaw: The Life and Times of William S. Burroughs* by T. Morgan. Copyright © 1991 by T. Morgan. Published by Pimlico/Random House. **22** From "Miracle Skipper Survives" by Rebecca Lang from *The Canberra Times*, December 29, 1993. Copyright © 1993 by *The Canberra Times*. **26** From "United States of America," p. 1248 of the *Cambridge Encyclopedia*. Copyright © 1990 by Cambridge University Press. Reprinted by permission. **35** From "You Can Get a Good Night's Rest" by Barbara Floria from *Vitality*, August 1994. Copyright © 1994 by *Vitality*. Reprinted by permission. **60** The Boston Phone Directory, p. 19. Copyright © 1995 NYNEX Information Resources Company. Reprinted by permission of NYNEX Information Resources Company. **68** Adapted from Oxfam. Advertisement used courtesy of Oxfam Hong Kong. **82** From "Tinker, Tailor, Paleontologist or Hairdresser?" by Deborah Holder, *The Independent on Sunday*, April 10, 1994. Copyright © 1994 by Newspaper Publishing PLC, London. Reprinted by permission. **86** From "Voices Across America" in USA Today, July 13, 1993. Copyright © 1993 by the Roper Center for Public Opinion Research. Reprinted by permission. **97** From "The Same Old Life" by Kenneth A. Walston from *Vitality*, June 1994. Copyright © 1994 by *Vitality*. Reprinted by permission.

Irregular Verb Chart

SIMPLE FORM ►	PAST FORM ►	PAST PARTICIPLE	SIMPLE FORM ►	PAST FORM ►	PAST PARTICIPLE
arise	arose	arisen	let	let	let
be	was	been	light	lit	lit
begin	began	begun	lose	lost	lost
bite	bit	bitten	make	made	made
blow	blew	blown	mean	meant	meant
break	broke	broken	meet	met	met
bring	brought	brought	pay	paid	paid
build	built	built	put	put	put
buy	bought	bought	read	read	read
catch	caught	caught	ride	rode	ridden
choose	chose	chosen	ring	rang	rung
cost	cost	cost	run	ran	run
cut	cut	cut	say	said	said
do	did	done	see	saw	seen
draw	drew	drawn	sell	sold	sold
drink	drank	drunk	send	sent	sent
drive	drove	driven	shoot	shot	shot
eat	ate	eaten	show	showed	shown
fall	fell	fallen	shut	shut	shut
feed	fed	fed	sing	sang	sung
feel	felt	felt	sink	sank	sunk
fight	fought	fought	sit	sat	sat
find	found	found	sleep	slept	slept
fly	flew	flown	speak	spoke	spoken
forget	forgot	forgotten	stand	stood	stood
get	got	gotten	swim	swam	swum
give	gave	given	take	took	taken
go	went	gone	teach	taught	taught
grow	grew	grown	tell	told	told
have	had	had	think	thought	thought
hear	heard	heard	throw	threw	thrown
hold	held	held	understand	understood	understood
keep	kept	kept	wake	woke	woken
know	knew	known	wear	wore	worn
learn	learned	learned	win	won	won
leave	left	left	write	wrote	written

Student Tapescript

Unit 1 Celebrations

Tasks 2 a, 2 b, 2 c, Conversation 1, page 10

Questioner: How long have you lived in Australia, Jack?

Jack: I moved from Baltimore to Adelaide, Australia, about eight years ago. The most important festival here is the Festival of Arts they have every two years, beginning on March 1st. It's great, really; they cater to every taste in music, art, literature, and theater. And they have performers from all over the world. I've seen some great stuff over the years, including a play directed by the Italian film maker Antonioni. I've also seen the Bolshoi Ballet and the Boston Symphony Orchestra.

Conversation 2, page 10

A: How was Rio, Paula?

B: Wild. I've been there a few times, but never for Carnival. Everything they say about it is true and then some.

A: What do you mean?

B: Well, there's this fantastic parade, and people never sleep, and there's nonstop music and dancing. I tell you, the Brazilians have to be the most exciting people on earth.

A: Yes, but what's the festival for?

B: What's it for?

A: Yes, what's it supposed to be celebrating?

B: Who knows? Who cares? The only ones who miss out are the clothing manufacturers!

Conversation 3, page 10

Suriwong: My name is Suriwong, and I'll be your host on today's tour. Before we leave the hotel, I should tell you that today is Loy Kratong, the Water Festival. It's an important Buddhist religious festival, but tourists remember it because they usually get wet.

Person 1: Wet?

S: Yes, you soon know it's a water festival because young people use it as an excuse to throw water on people. You'll see them all over the city with buckets of water. So I suggest that if you're wearing good clothes or expensive jewelry, you go back to your room and change before we leave. You definitely get wet!

Person 2: Even though we're on a tour bus.

S: Sure. The kids will jump onto the bus and start throwing water.

Conversation 4, page 10

I'm Nina French from Universal Travel. This week's special is a return trip to Hong Kong in mid-June for the Dragon Boat Festival. It's one of the most important festivals on the religious calendar, but it's also lots of fun. Prices include transfers, round-trip airfares, and five nights' shared accommodations. Call Universal Travel now at 555-5832 to reserve your spot!

Unit 1, Tasks 2 a and 2 b, Interview 1, page 13

Interviewer: Hi! I'm interviewing celebrities about their birthdays. I have just a few questions to ask you, Mariel.

Mariel: Shoot.

I: What's the best birthday present you ever received?

M: In 1975 I got a baby doll made of that lovely, soft plastic stuff. And I still have her, though her eyes are gone and her hair is all pulled out.

I: What would make the perfect birthday gift for you?

M: Nothing! Birthdays make me sick. I have a hard time accepting gifts, and, besides, I never get those very expensive books on art, photography, and film. They're all I want.

I: How do you choose gifts for other people?

M: I don't, usually. It's silly to buy presents for adult friends and relatives. I prefer to have a party and cook delicious food for people. I make an exception for kids, and give lots of toys to my nieces and nephews.

I: How much do you spend?

M: A lot, as much as I can! I spoil them rotten so they'll like me more!

Interview 2, page 13

Interviewer: Natasha, what's the best birthday present you ever received?

Natasha: Anything involving travel. When I was nine, my parents took us on an Italian cruise ship. I'll never forget watching Italian films in the ship's cinema and seeing my parents dancing in the bar.

I: What would be the perfect gift for next year?

N: Mmm, what I would really love is a massage—a year's supply would be ideal.

I: How do you choose gifts for other people?

N: I tend to see something that reminds me of the person and buy it. Then I wait for an appropriate occasion to give them the gift. I like to give things I know they would never treat themselves to.

I: How much do you spend?

N: Not much. It's the thought that counts, not the cost.

Interview 3, page 13

Interviewer: What's the best birthday present you ever received, Rod?

Rod: I've loved everything I've ever received except socks and underwear.

I: What would be the perfect gift?

R: A fun-filled, exciting year ahead.

I: How do you choose gifts for other people?

R: Oh, I don't know—I guess if I know that they like something, or if they've asked for it.

I: How much do you spend?

R: Whatever it takes, as long as the person is happy with it.

Unit 1, Task 1, page 15

Jim: Hello, Tomoko?

Tomoko: Oh, hi, Jim.

J: I'm calling to see if you can come to my birthday party on Saturday night.

T: I can't, sorry. I'm having dinner with a friend.

J: Would you be able to come later?

T: Well, I guess I could come around eleven. Would you mind if I brought my friend?

J: No, not at all. See you then.

Unit 2 Believe It or Not

Tasks 2 a, 2 b, and 2 c, page 18

Pete: I had a really weird thing happen to me last night.

Mark: Yeah? What was that, Pete?

P: Well, I was relaxing at home watching TV, and I had this strange feeling something was wrong.

Gina: What do you mean, wrong?

P: Hang on, Gina, and I'll tell you—it was, like, this really uncomfortable feeling. I can't explain it really. I tried to ignore it for a while, but in the end I had to do something. I have an elderly neighbor, and I had a feeling that something was wrong. I just had this feeling that I had to go check on her. I have a key to her apartment because I often do her shopping for her, so I can let myself in. Anyway, I went and knocked on the door, and there was no answer, and I called out a couple of times and there was still no answer, so I let myself in, and there she was lying on the floor.

M: Not . . .

P: No, she was OK. Well, not OK—she'd fallen and broken her hip. But, like I say, it was weird. I called the ambulance and stayed with her, and she said she'd been hoping someone would come to see her. She said she'd been thinking that if someone didn't come, she'd die there on the floor of her apartment.

G: That's called telepathy.

P: What? Did you say telepathy?

G: Yeah, telepathy—when people can read each other's thoughts. She was sending out mental messages, and you picked them up.

M: Come on, you don't believe that stuff, do you?

G: I'm not sure.

P: After what happened to me last night, I believe it, I can tell you.

M: Well, I don't believe a word of it—I think it's nonsense. What about you, Gina?

G: I'm really not sure, Mark. I think there's something to it. When I was younger, my brother and I used to play this game. One of us used to think of a number and write it on a piece of paper and then concentrate real hard on the number, and the other one would concentrate, too, and then write down the number that came into his head.

M: And?

G: Well, it didn't work all the time, but most of the time it did—like seven out of ten times when we compared the numbers they were the same. A little scary, really.

M: It's just a coincidence.

P: You're just a skeptic, Mark.

Task 2 c, page 22

Well, when the wave hit the boat, my safety harness broke and I was swept overboard. I don't really understand how it happened, but it did. I heard someone yell out, but then my boat, *Wild One*, went off into the darkness and I was alone in a very rough sea. I then spent five and a half hours in the water. The place where it happened was, oh, about 50 kilometers from shore. It was likely that I wouldn't see another day, but I always thought I'd beat the odds. At first I was watching out for *Wild One*. The rest of the crew knew I was gone, so they were sure to come back and look for me. After a while, I saw the boat's lights when it came looking for me. They were within about 300 meters of me, but the spotlight just missed me. The reason why they didn't see me was because of the huge waves. You know, I started sailing when I was seven, and started ocean racing when I was about eighteen, but I'd never been overboard before. I believed I was going to survive, but it was very cold, and as the hours passed I started to get desperate—and frozen! It was around 5 A.M. when I saw the lights of a tanker coming towards me. I figured it was probably my last chance. At first, I thought they were going to miss me, and then they made a slight turn and I yelled out "Help!" and they heard me. Then another yacht appeared. These guys were terrific. They gave me dry clothes, and then one just jumped into the bunk and hung onto me.

They covered us with as much dry clothing as they could, and the guy in with me stayed to transfer his body heat to me.

Unit 3 Origins

Tasks 4 a and 4 b, page 27

There are many reasons why people emigrate. Poverty, hunger, and hardship are major reasons, and there are many examples throughout history of mass migration brought about by these factors. Hunger drove many people out of Ireland in the 1850s, for example. The desire to escape from political persecution is also an important reason for people to leave the land of their birth. In the 1920s, this was the reason why many people escaped from the former Soviet Union. A desire to escape from the chaos and heartache of war has also been a major cause of population movement in many parts of the world. After the Second World War, millions of people left war-torn Europe for New World countries such as Canada and the United States. More recently, people have left places such as Cyprus and Lebanon for the same reason. On the positive side, opportunities for a better life in a new country attract many people. In the 1950s and 1960s millions of people were attracted to Australia, a country that wanted to increase its population quickly. These people wanted a better future for their children. Uncertainty about the future is another important reason why people emigrate. During the early 1990s, many people left Hong Kong because they were uncertain about what the future might hold after the British colony returned to China after 1997.

Task 1, page 28

A: Why did you decide to go to Japan?

B: I've always been fascinated by Japanese culture and I've read a lot about the country and its people, and I wanted to see it for myself.

A: And what did you think?

B: Well, it was the most incredible experience I've ever had.

Tasks 2 a, 2 b, and 2 d, page 29

Anne: Whenever I meet new people in this country I always have to explain where I'm from, whereas when I'm back in Britain, I'm surrounded by people who know about my background—friends, family, and relatives are always around. When I first moved to Australia, I felt I had to explain my background to everyone I met because I came from a culture where everyone likes to know where you fit in. I got sick of it after a while.

Denise: I think that's your British background, Anne, 'cause I don't feel that way living in California. People are coming and going all the time, so they don't care that much about where you're from. They might say "Where're you from? Oh, Australia," and then they'll ask about kangaroos or something and then that's it.

Dave: Well, a lot of times I feel really ignorant, especially about popular culture. You go somewhere and everybody knows someone's name—a famous actor or singer or whatever—who's known only in Australia. I found it time and time again when I first moved from Canada—everybody knew about someone or some event, but I didn't have a clue.

A: Right.

D: Well, that doesn't happen in California, 'cause California is the world's culture.

Any person who's popular in California is going to be popular everywhere else 'cause they're going to be marketed everywhere else.

Task 1, page 31

Australian: What makes Canada special for you Dave?

Dave: I guess it's the tolerance of the people that makes the place special for me. What also makes it special is the mix of nationalities. We have people here from all over the world. What about you?

A: Well, what makes Australia special is that it's at the end of the earth, so it's still relatively innocent. I guess it's also the mix of people from all over the world. I guess we're a bit like Canada from that perspective.

Unit 4 Good Advice

Task 2, page 33

I know that I'm considered a little bit odd by my friends—I mean, I'm the only one who does it. But then I'm in a position to do it because I work from home, so it's not a big deal. But then, I'm not all that unusual, you know. Some of the most famous people of this century used to do it. John F. Kennedy used to love a quick one in the afternoons—whenever he got the chance, he'd slip out of the Oval Office for thirty minutes of bliss. Some of my friends think it's decadent, but I don't. I mean, I stay up late at night working, so why not? A quick half-hour nap and I feel fresh and rested for the rest of the day and evening.

Tasks 2 b, 2 c, and 2 d, page 34

Josie: Hi, Tessie.

Tessie: Oh, hi, Josie.

J: Gee, you look terrible.

T: I feel terrible. I've been working hard, and I haven't had a decent night's sleep in ages.

J: Well, you need to get a good night's rest, or your day will be a waste.

T: Tell me about it! I just don't know what to do. I've had a lot of stress at work lately, and . . .

J: And as soon as you go to bed, you start thinking about work, right?

T: Right.

J: Well, what you should do is set aside some worry or planning time early in the evening. If you do that, then you'll have all your worrying out of the way before you go to bed, and you won't be going over all your problems once your head hits the pillow. Do you go to bed at the same time every night?

T: No, I don't. What with friends, family, and house guests, I never know what time I'll get to bed.

J: Mmm, well, if you get to bed at a regular time, your body will get into a pattern and you'll sleep better. What about exercise?

T: Not often, I'm afraid. Tennis once a month or so, and a walk in the park on the weekend.

J: If you can take a thirty-minute walk, jog, or swim three or four times a week, that'll help you sleep, too. And of course you should never have a large heavy meal or drink coffee before you go to bed. In fact, if you drink coffee within eight hours of going to bed it can interfere with your sleep.

T: I never eat a large meal in the evening, but I do drink coffee.

J: Well, that's part of your problem.

T: My, you're a real gold mine of information, Josie. How come you know so much?

J: Well, I'm a poor sleeper too, so I read articles on how to get better sleep.

T: And it works?

J: Not really, but it helps pass the time!

Task 1, page 36

A: My sister and her husband are coming to visit this weekend.

B: Oh, that's great!

A: Well, it's good and bad. She's very messy, and he's an insomniac.

B: A *what*?

A: An insomniac—someone who has trouble sleeping. He spends most of the night watching TV and keeping everyone else awake.

B: Oh, no.

A: What should I do if she leaves her stuff all over the place?

B: If she leaves her clothes all over the place, you should put them in a bag and send them to the most expensive cleaner in town.

A: What a great idea! And what should I do when her husband keeps us all awake?

B: When you go to bed, take the TV remote control with you.

A: What a great idea!

Tasks 2 a, 2 b, and 2 c, page 38

A: Right now we have Camilla on the line. How can we help you, Camilla?

B: Well, I'm calling up about my daughter, who's a chronic nail-biter. I've tried everything, including putting that horrible-tasting stuff on her nails, but nothing seems to work.

C: You know, Camilla, I had the same problem with one of my sons, and what we did was to give him a dollar at the start of each week, and we then took a dime away every time he bit his nails. At the end of the week we let him keep the money that was left over.

B: And it worked?

C: Well, I must admit that he still bites his nails at times but not nearly as much.

B: OK, well, I guess I'll try it.

A: Thanks, Camilla. That next person on the line is Tom.

D: Hi there. I have a really big problem with junk food. I just can't help myself. I've tried those appetite-suppressing pills, but they're expensive, and they just don't seem to work.

B: You know, Tom, this is really a common problem. I suggest you check to see if there's a branch of Overeaters Anonymous in your neighborhood. They're a voluntary group and give great support.

D: Did you say Overeaters Anonymous?

C: That's right. They exist in most cities.

D: OK, thanks a lot.

A: Next we have one of our younger listeners—Melissa.

C: How can we help you, Melissa?

E: My little brother always makes weird noises when he's reading or doing homework. It drives me crazy. I tell my parents, but they say I should ignore it. How can I make him stop?

C: Is he aware that he's making these noises?

E: I don't know. I don't think he is.

C: Well, why not try tape-recording him when he makes the noises and then playing the tape back. That should make him realize how annoying it is.

E: Hey, that's a great idea! Thanks.

A: Thank you, Melissa.

Task 1, page 39

Mitch: You moved back in with your folks after college, didn't you, Lisa?

Lisa: Yes, I did.

M: How's it working out?

L: Oh, fine. We have our moments, though.

M: What do you mean?

L: Well, my brothers Bradley and Stu are still living at home, and they're both kind of crazy guys.

M: Kind of crazy, huh? In what way?

L: Well, they both have really weird habits. Bradley's a real slob. He leaves his junk all over the house—it's a pit. And he smokes in the house.

M: And Stu?

L: Stu's into noise. Music, video, TV, everything has to be at 1,000 decibels, He never seems to sleep—says he can't, but then he keeps everyone else awake.

M: So if you had to choose one of your brothers to room with, who would it be?

L: Oh, well, I hate smokers. I like people who are neat, and I don't like people whose idea of a good time is to stay up late and make a lot of noise. So if I had to choose, well, I guess I'd live alone! Or live with someone who's away most of the time. How about you?

M: I like people who think of others, you know, whose attitude is considerate. I don't like people who think only of themselves. I'd live only with someone who's going to help with the housework and basically keep to themselves.

Communication Challenge 4 a, page 113

The most irritating person I ever lived with was a college friend—or ex-friend. He was my best pal in college, but we didn't stay pals for long—not once we started living together. Oh, he had his good points and his bad points. He was very neat, always did the dishes, and would even offer to do my laundry. Unfortunately, as far as I'm concerned, his bad habits outweighed his good ones. He wasn't at all interested in decent food, and used to live off TV dinners and stuff like that. When it was his turn to cook, I had to eat frozen peas and instant mashed potatoes. Yuk. And he had awful taste in music. Pop music, which I hate. At least he didn't play it loudly, but he was an insomniac, so he'd stay up late at night and keep me up, too. When he wasn't listening to pop music, he was watching sports on TV. As far as I'm concerned, he's the sort of person only a mother could love.

The most annoying person I know is my kid brother. Whenever I have friends around, he wants to be included in whatever we're doing. He's three years younger than I am, and our interests are very different, but that doesn't stop him. He thinks he's missing out on something if he's not included. And if I shut him out of my room, he makes so much noise that I can't hear myself think! He's OK in some ways, and if I'm ever sick or anything he's very sweet and sympathetic, but mostly he's a pain.

What irritates me about my wife? Well, she's always right—at least she thinks she is—and I'm always wrong. That's definitely her most irritating habit. I wish she'd stop smoking—although she doesn't smoke inside the apartment, thank goodness. There's no question that her good points outweigh her bad points. She's always thinking of others—that's probably her best point. Every Sunday, she visits her elderly aunt and uncle to see how they are and if they need anything. And she always remembers people's birthdays—unlike me.

My brother's wife moved in with our family after they got married, and she drives me nuts. She's incredibly neat—always putting my stuff away for me. She can't stand to see things left lying around. And she always goes to bed early—around 9:30, and after that time it's impossible to have music playing or the TV on. Oh, yeah, and the other thing is that she sees herself as a great cook, so we have to eat these gourmet meals all the time—Italian or French, mostly. I haven't had any decent junk food since she came to live with us.

Unit 5 Review Unit

Tasks 3 a and 3 b, Conversation 1, pages 41 and 42

A: So, what do you think I should do, Bob?

Bob: Well, you're in luck, actually, because the Downtown Bus Company has just started a new service from the train terminal and it goes past your office building. So you could get the subway and then take a bus.

A: That's great! It'll really solve my problem.

B: Oh, and there's one other thing.

A: What's that?

B: Well, in the future, don't share a ride with someone who's thinking of taking a new job.

Conversation 2, pages 41 and 42

Female: I've tried talking to him, but it hasn't done any good at all. He's the kind of person who doesn't listen. It disrupts the whole household, but he doesn't seem to care.

A: It's a problem that he won't consider other people's feelings.

F: I don't know what to do. It's particularly hard on my younger son, who's studying for his final exams at the moment. I mean, last night it was after one o'clock when he came home and put the music on.

A: Why don't you put the chain on the door? Lock him out for the night. He'll get the message.

Conversation 3, pages 41 and 42

A: So, do you think you can help me out?

B: I'm not sure. I've never met anyone like that before.

A: Yeah, well, she's the only one I know. And she had to invite me to her birthday party!

B: Actually, I know what you can get her.

A: What's that?

B: One of those cards that say "For the person who has everything!"

A: And that's all?

B: That's all!

Conversation 4, pages 41 and 42

A: I can't stand to go home at night—the place is such a dump.

B: I had the same problem with my roommate last year. It got really bad when I started my new job, because I couldn't find any of my stuff. I was late every morning.

A: And what did you do?

B: Well, I tried talking to her, but she doesn't realize she's like that. Luckily, I solved the problem just in time.

A: You did? How?

B: I threw all her stuff out the window. She shaped up real fast!

Unit 6 That's a Smart Idea

Tasks 2 a, 2 c, and 2 d, Interview Part 1, pages 44 and 45

Nicholas: Good evening and welcome to *Ideas*, the arts program for all ages. Tonight I'm talking to Roger Scott and Ingrid Gould, two of the most creative people in Canada. The subject of tonight's discussion is the nature of creativity and the creative process. I'd like to know how you two go about creating your work. Roger?

Roger: Yes, thanks, Nicholas. This is the first question I get asked in interviews. How do you go about it? Is it divine inspiration, or is it a whole lot of hard work? Well, in my case it's a lot of difficult, analytical work, with a little inspiration thrown in from time to time. I have some basic ideas about what I want to communicate, and I write them down, and then it's a process of working on them laboriously—writing and rewriting, showing the stuff to people I trust—until I'm satisfied. I mean, you're never really satisfied, but eventually you have to say to yourself, well, this is as good as it's going to get. And sometimes you'll work all day, go to bed, get up the next day, decide it's all rubbish, and throw it away and start again—then work all night!

N: Sounds like really hard work.

R: It is!

N: And what about you, Ingrid, do you work in the same way?

Ingrid: Well, no, actually. It's interesting—sometimes I sit and stare at the page for hours, and it's blank at the end of the day.

R: Same here.

I: But with me it's a much more holistic kind of thing. I mean, I don't assemble the bits and pieces like Roger. I think he's much more logical and analytical than I am. I tend to work in a more impulsive and intuitive way. As I say, one day there'll be nothing; then the next day I'll get up and it just flows from somewhere. It's a strange and mysterious process.

Interview Part 2, pages 44 and 45

N: So, although you're both creative writers, you work in very different ways.

I: I guess so, although I wouldn't want you to get the idea that it's all inspiration on my part. True, the ideas might come to me all at once—you know, the light-bulb effect—but that doesn't mean there isn't a lot of hard work as well. Someone once said that being a poet is ten percent inspiration and ninety percent perspiration. I guess with me it's maybe twenty percent inspiration and eighty percent perspiration. It's great when things do flow well. The last poem I wrote was great; the words just flowed out of the ends of my fingers. I thought, wow, where did this come from—it had come from somewhere, but sometimes even I don't know!

R: And, of course, for me it's different because I have to work with the people who write the music. So I might have what I think are wonderful words, but they don't fit the music, so they have to be rewritten.

N: Tough.

R: Yeah, tough.

Tasks 3 a and 3 d, page 48

A: I have this amazing aunt. She's always coming up with crazy ideas.

B: Oh, yeah? Like what?

A: All kinds of things. Like, a few years ago, she was obsessed over the fact that socks were always getting lost in the wash—you know how washing machines will "eat" half of a pair of socks?

B: Yeah.

A: So Aunt Josephine bought some strips of Velcro and sewed them around the cuff of each sock. The idea was that you just touch them together before throwing them into the wash, and they'll come out together.

B: Brilliant!

A: Yes, except that no one in the family would wear them.

B: Why not?

A: They had all kinds of objections. Cousin Danielle said that if the Velcro toughed her skirt when she was sitting in class and the teacher asked her to stand up, it would pull her skirt down. (*B's laughter*) And Uncle Todd said that if he crossed his legs at the ankles the socks would stick, and when he stood up, he'd fall flat on his face. Cousin Lou said that it wouldn't help him 'cause he didn't have any matching socks anyway! (*A's and B's laughter*)

B: Well, she tried.

A: Yeah, it was a neat idea.

Unit 7 Creatures Great and Small

Task 2 a, page 51

Question 1: The dodo is (A) an extinct animal; (B) a make-believe creature; (C) a living animal.

Question 2: The giant panda is an endangered animal. True or false?

Question 3: Kangaroos are considered gourmet food in Australia. True or false?

Question 4: Elephants are used as working animals in (A) Thailand; (B) Australia; (C) Taiwan.

Question 5: Kiwis are (A) small horses; (B) birds; (C) make-believe creatures.

Question 6: Elderly people who have pets tend to live longer than those who live alone. True or false?

Task 2, page 52

A: I'm afraid I just don't believe it.

B: Well, it's true, according to this TV show I saw the other day. The owner had spent about 15 years teaching him how to do it. It was fascinating. I mean, he was able to do a lot more than simply follow instructions and say "hello"—when I was a kid, we had one who could do that. This one could also describe things and could even communicate his feelings. You could ask him to count things such as the number of plastic toys on a tray. He gave the wrong answer to one question and then apologized!

A: Did what?

B: Apologized. Said he was sorry. Another time he got frustrated and said, "I'm gonna go away" and turned his back.

A: Yes, but the question is—does he know what he's saying, or is "I'm gonna go away" just a bunch of sounds he makes when he's frustrated?

B: Oh, I think he knows very well what he's saying.

Task 2 a, page 55

A: Why did you decide to become a naturalist?

B: Oh, simple. I find the natural world so much more interesting than the human world.

A: Seriously?

B: Seriously. It's precious, it's beautiful, it's magical, it's exciting, it's dramatic. Shall I go on?

A: I think we get the idea.

B: You know, I'm not that interested in watching humans hunt, but when I discovered a hunting spider that spins an elastic web and actually throws it to capture its food—well, I find that the most dramatic thing I've ever seen.

A: What's the most incredible thing you've ever seen?

B: I'd have to say the Christmas Island land crabs.

A: The Christmas Island land crabs?

B: Yes. You know, we can sit here in Florida and look at the calendar and say, "When the moon is in the third quarter on July 27th we'll go to the Christmas Islands and on that day, five million crabs will come out of the forest and go into the sea, just like they've been doing for ten million years.

A: That *is* incredible.

B: And what's more, it's caused by the moon, and the tides, and the earth.

A: What's the most difficult trip you've ever made?

B: Oh, that would have to be a trip I took to Australia many years ago. I wanted to film the tree kangaroo in the tropical rain forests of northern Queensland. In those days, travel was a real adventure. It took me four weeks. Nobody had heard of the place. There were no planes going there, not even ships. But it was lots of fun. Now, of course, the tree kangaroos are an endangered species.

Unit 8 Communications

Task 3, Conversation 1, page 61

Male: Reckitt and Fixx. How may I help you?

Female: I'd like to speak to the Marketing Manager, please.

M: Putting you through now. *(ringing sound)* I'm sorry, she doesn't seem to be at that number; I'll just . . .

F: Please hurry.

M: Excuse me?

F: Please hurry. I'm calling from Argentina—and I'm on a public phone.

M: Let me try her at another number.

Conversation 2, page 61

Female: So, how's it going over there on the west coast?

Nancy: Great. The weather's fantastic; there are so many things to do—I haven't had a spare moment since I got here. And the new job's wonderful.

F: Great! Hey, listen . . .

N: And I'm a continent away from that creep, Jim.

Jim: Hi, Nancy!

N: Who's that?

J: It's Jim.

F: I was trying to tell you this was a conference call.

Conversation 3, page 61

A: Marcia, you still there?

B: Yes, I am.

A: Sorry about that, it was the dental clinic. They want to change my appointment again, can you believe it?

B: Oh, they're always doing that—same thing happened to me last week.

A: Anyway, as I was saying, next week Rob's going to Seattle on business. Do you want to have dinner . . . *(click from call waiting)* Oh, sorry, can you hold on a sec? That might be him.

Task 3, page 63

A: What do you do, Clive?

B: I'm a communications consultant.

A: A communications consultant? What's that?

B: It's someone who advises companies on every aspect of communications, both within the company and in its dealings with the outside world. It's fascinating stuff. Every aspect of a company says something about it.

A: Such as?

B: Such as where they're located. Such as the letterhead they use. Such as the furniture you find in the director's office. Such as corporate logos. These all send extremely powerful messages.

A: Logos are powerful?

B: Sure. It's interesting that *logo* is Greek for "word," yet most logos are pictures—they're pictures that deliver a message. As I've said, a logo can be a very powerful tool.

A: I'm not sure I'm with you—can you give me an example?

B: Sure. I was recently called in by the West-East Banking Corporation, a medium-sized firm on the west coast. They were trying to break into Asian markets and were having a tough time. They couldn't understand what the problem was. Two of their competitors were trying to get into Asian markets and doing very well at it. So I looked at their marketing strategy, their promotional literature, and so on, and saw right away what the problem was.

A: And?

B: It basically had to do with their corporate logo.

A: What was wrong with their logo?

B: Well, their logo was an owl. What does an owl signify to you?

A: Wisdom, of course—the wise old owl.

B: Right. In many Asian cultures, however, it symbolizes sneakiness. It has the same sort of image as the cunning fox. So, this logo was sending exactly the opposite message than the one they wanted.

A: Fascinating. So they changed their logo?

B: They changed their logo, and the problem was solved. There are other aspects to a corporate image, of course—it's not *just* the logo; it's the symbolism behind the logo.

What's the first word that comes into your mind when I say "Deep Springs Mineral Water"?

A: Oh, I don't know—um, freshness, purity.

B: Purity. Exactly. And do you remember what happened to Deep Springs a few years ago?

A: Oh, there was some kind of scandal, wasn't there?

B: Not a scandal, exactly. A few of their bottles were found to have impurities in them. It was critically important, because of their corporate image of purity. What did they do? They immediately withdrew all of their products. But then, more importantly, the chief executives called a conference with key journalists and explained what was going on. Because they were up-front about it, they got extremely good press and were saved as a business. They saved their image as well.

Unit 9 Helping Hands

Tasks 2 a, 2 b, and 2 c, Conversation 1, pages 68 and 69

Linda: Excuse me.

Man: Yes?

L: I wonder if I could talk to you for a few minutes.

M: Well, I . . .

L: My name is Linda, and I work for Educare. Here's my ID card. And here's some literature.

M: I'm sorry, I'm busy right now, and . . .

L: I just want you to take a quick look; it'll only take a minute.

M: I really don't have the time right now.

L: But this is really important. It's an educational support plan so kids from poor backgrounds can finish high school. It's an extremely worthy cause, and all you have to do is commit to $300 a year—that's less than $10 a week! And it'll help give a kid the chance to . . .

M: I've really got to run.

L: Oh, OK, thanks for your time.

Conversation 2, pages 68 and 69

Male 1: Hello.

Male 2: Good morning. My name is Mike, and I'm calling on behalf of the Everett Foundation.

M1: The?

M2: Everett Foundation. We're a registered charity, and we . . .

M1: Are you raising money?

M2: Well, I . . .

M1: How did you get my number?

M2: Well, we . . .

M1: I really resent you people invading my privacy like this. If you want to solicit from people, you should knock on doors. I want you to tell the head of your organization that I disapprove.

M2: Certainly, sir. But I just want to take a few minutes of your time to tell you about our foundation. We raise money for AIDS education.

M1: And I suppose you get a commission, eh?

M2: Well, yes, as a registered charity worker, I do this on a commission basis. There's nothing wrong with . . .

M1: I think it's disgusting, and it's exploitation. I must say I disapprove of all this charity stuff. I worked hard for my money, and I intend to keep it. Good bye. *(Phone slams.)*

Conversation 3, pages 68 and 69

Female 1: Hi.

Female 2: Hi. I hope I'm not bothering you. My name's Martha, and I wonder if you could take a look at this brochure.

F1: Are you looking for donations?

F2: Well, yes, the Blue Star Charity Appeal. You might've seen our ad on TV.

F1: No, I don't think I did. You know, my son always tells me not to . . .

F2: Well, this is a really good cause. We do volunteer work in a number of Third World countries. We're non-profit, non-religious, and we work on a volunteer basis. It's all in the brochure.

F1: Hmm. OK, then. How much would you like?

F2: Whatever you'd like to give!

Conversation 4, pages 68 and 69

Male 1: Good morning, my name's Peter. My badge here shows that I'm collecting for the World Youth Fund.

Male 2: The World Youth Fund? Yeah, I've heard of it, but what does it do?

M1: Well, it's a fund established to promote international understanding among the young. Here's a brochure. And I'd like you to think about giving some money.

M2: Yes, it looks like an interesting cause. We could do with a little more international understanding these days.

M1: That's what we think.

M2: And how much do people usually give?

M1: Well, anything from five to five hundred dollars.

M2: Is it tax deductible?

M1: Oh, sure. I can give you a receipt and everything.

M2: OK, well, I'll give you thirty dollars. How's that?

M1: That's very generous! It'll be very much appreciated, I can tell you.

Tasks 2 a and 2 b, page 71

Interviewer: You have an interesting job, then, Harry.

Harry: I guess I do.

I: Could you tell us about it?

H: Well, the official title is Assistant Guest Relations Manager.

I: Here at the Pacific Hotel?

H: Right. But my unofficial title is Harry the Helper.

I: Harry the Helper?

H: Uh-huh.

I: And how did you come by such a title?

H: Well, it started years ago. I was assistant to the night manager in those days, and one night—it was pretty quiet around here back then, believe it or not. Anyway, one night there was this terrible shouting coming from one of the rooms. I was the only one at the front desk, and I wasn't supposed to leave it, but this shouting just went on and on, and finally I went to see what was going on.

I: And what did you find?

H: The noise was coming from the VIP suite. We had a very important person in there.

I: The VIP?

H: Exactly. Anyway, this person—and I can't reveal the name—was taking a bath, and he got his big toe stuck up the spout of the faucet.

I: He what?

H: Had his toe stuck in the faucet.

I: How on earth . . . ?

H: He never said. And I never asked. Said he'd been trying to get it out for half an hour before he starting yelling for help. I tried pulling his foot, but it was wedged in there tight. We tried everything—soap, you name it. By this time the guy's embarrassment had worn off, and he was getting really upset. Then I had an idea. Earlier in the evening, I'd been using a special lubricant that comes in a spray can to fix squeaky doors. So I got some of this stuff and sprayed it all around his toe and on the faucet and stuff . . .

I: . . . and?

H: It did the trick. Toe came right out like a cork out of a bottle. It was pretty beat up, but it was still attached to the end of the foot!

I: And if you hadn't had your great idea?

H: If I hadn't had my great idea, he'd have been stuck in the tub all night. I guess we'd have had to call the fire department. Anyway, it worked out well for me. He gave me a tip equal to a week's pay, and called me Harry the Helper, and the name stuck.

I: And what other help have you given?

H: Oh, it varies from big things to small. Had a guy in once who was getting married, and he'd ripped his pin-striped pants right down the seam. This was about ten minutes before he was due in church.

I: And what did you do?

H: Well, we were about the same size, so I took off my own pants and lent them to him.

I: Right then and there?

H: Yes, if I hadn't, he would've missed his wedding. Who knows if he'd ever have gotten married.

I: And what other helping hand have you lent? Anything involving a celebrity?

H: Well, there was the time that the famous film star wandered into the lobby wearing nothing but a nightgown.

I: Really? What did you do?

H: Well, I realized right away that she was sleepwalking, and that it was important not to wake her up.

I: So?

H: So, I took her gently by the arm and led her back to her room. She never knew what happened.

I: And if you hadn't stepped in . . .

H: If I hadn't stepped in, she'd have ended up in the street!

I: So everyone thinks that you're a great helper.

H: Well, not quite everyone.

I: No?

H: No. My wife says that I'm no help at all around the house.

Unit 10 Review Unit

Task 3 a, page 76

Invention 1

Inventor: Well, I was at an international conference of inventors, and I was staying in this hotel, and I was taking a bath. Anyway, I finished my bath and . . .

Interviewer: . . . and you couldn't get the plug out.

Inventor: I couldn't get the plug out. Exactly. So I happened to notice the shampoo container hanging on the shower—you know, they have a big plastic hanging loop.

Interviewer: Uh, huh.

Inventor: And, I thought, well, if it had a big loop like the shampoo container, I'd be able to get it out. So that's how the Super-Loop Plug came about.

Invention 2

A: I think the most useful invention in recent years is the Post-it® Note.

B: The what?

A: The Post-it® Note. You know those little yellow notepads that have a strip of non-permanent adhesive on the back?

B: Oh, yeah.

A: Apparently the guy who invented it was trying to make a regular glue—you know, that would stick permanently. The stuff he came up with wouldn't stick, and he was about to throw it out when he had this great idea—that there are times when you don't want stuff to stick permanently. I use them to make notes on my books when I'm studying. Then when I've finished, I can remove the notes, and I don't have writing all over my books.

Invention 3

Interviewer: So what prompted you to come up with this ingenious invention?

Inventor: Well, I got sick of having these hooks that would fall off the wall. I'd get back to our apartment at night and go into the bathroom, and the towels would be all over the floor—and the same in the kitchen. The stick-on hooks just wouldn't stick.

Interviewer: And you didn't want to screw them to the wall?

Inventor: No, I didn't want unsightly holes in the wall. So I got this idea of using suction hooks when I was playing archery with my son. He has one of these archery sets with arrows that have suction cups on the end.

Interviewer: Brilliant.

Inventor: Yes. My husband said they'd never work, but they do. They stay on the wall until you want to move them, and when you want to move them it's easy and they don't leave holes or marks.

Unit 11 Speaking Personally

Task 3 a, page 78

Questioner: Mark, what do you enjoy doing more than anything else?

Mark: Oh, gosh. I think . . . playing the banjo.

Q: Yeah? OK. What's your greatest ambition in life?

M: To be as good a banjo player as Doc Boggs, the famous musician from Kentucky.

Q: What's your greatest achievement so far?

M: Umm, I think my greatest achievement so far has been learning how to write computer programs.

Q: Who do you admire most in the world, and why?

M: Living?

Q: Yeah.

M: Oh, um, I don't really know. I admire how Doc Boggs plays the banjo.

Q: OK. What's the best thing that's ever happened to you?

M: Probably the best thing is that I was able to buy a house in the mountains.

Q: Great. What's the most exciting thing that's ever happened to you?

M: Most exciting thing? Er, I guess traveling to India must rate pretty highly as an exciting thing.

Questioner: Vanessa, what do you enjoy doing more than anything else?

Vanessa: Oh, writing stories.

Q: Writing stories? What kind of stories?

V: Short stories.

Q: Have any been published?

V: No, not yet.

Q: OK. What's your greatest ambition in life?

V: To be happy and successful.

Q: What is your greatest achievement so far?

V: I'd have to say getting my present job. Yeah.

Q: What is your job?

V: Designer and editor. And considering two years ago I didn't think I'd be anywhere, and here I am, feeling successful and learning lots of new skills.

Q: Who do you admire most in the world, and why?

V: Um, I'd have to say my mother. I know that sounds corny, but . . .

Q: Why?

V: Just because she's been through a lot, and she's survived it. And she's taught me a lot.

Q: What's the best thing that's ever happened to you?

V: I guess I'd have to say my job again.

Q: What's the most exciting thing that's ever happened to you?

V: I won twenty dollars at the horse races! *(laughs)* No, seriously, I suppose when I won a design competition in art school— yeah, that was the most exciting thing.

Questioner: Sylvia, what do you enjoy more than anything else?

Sylvia: Probably lying on a beach looking at the water and thinking of going in for a swim.

Q: Yeah? OK. What's your greatest ambition in life?

S: To do a little less work and to spend more time doing things I enjoy.

Q: What is your greatest achievement so far?

S: Learning to speak modern Greek.

Q: Who do you admire most in the world, and why?

S: Well, now, that's a hard one. Hmm. Probably a college professor I had once. She's got a wonderful, caring personality, and she's also done well in her career.

Q: What's the best thing that's ever happened to you?

S: Moving to Toronto.

Q: What's the most exciting thing that's ever happened to you?
S: Meeting Marilyn Horne.
Q: Who?
S: Marilyn Horne, the famous opera singer.

Tasks 2 a and 2 b, Conversation 1, page 81

Ellie

I wanted to be a flight attendant when I was very young because I saw a TV show about them. But then I realized what a tough job it was. I also wanted to be a graphic designer because a cool friend of my parents was one. But I took a graphics course at school and realized it wasn't what I thought it would be. The other day I saw a program about genetic engineering and got quite interested. I talked to my biology teacher about it. I'm good in science. So at the moment, that's what I plan to go into when I graduate.

Conversation 2, page 81

Charles

When I was a kid, I wanted to be a vet. We had lots of pets, and I was crazy about them. Ultimately, though, I think two things influenced me. My mother decided to have a fifth child—I was the fourth—so I spent a lot of my time between the ages of eleven and thirteen taking care of a baby. Then when I was sixteen one of my teachers suggested that I'd be good with emotionally disturbed kids, and I was hooked. I went to the local teachers college, and, so far, I love what I'm doing.

Conversation 3, page 81

Mary

I'm an only child. My father was a printer, and my mother taught me needlework. I never had much ambition—never thought about what I'd do when I grew up. Then one day my grandparents took me to the circus, and I knew that's what I wanted to do. For years, I was determined to join a circus as an acrobat or something. The fact that I had absolutely no talent never occurred to me. Then, in my teenage years, I was crazy about pop music and wanted to be a radio DJ. I even applied for a job at a radio station. Then, after all the silly dreams, I got out of school and started at Miller's Department Store, and I've been there for fifteen years. Funny how things turn out. It's OK, I guess, but I sometimes wonder what it would have been like in the circus.

Unit 12 Attitudes

Tasks 2 b, 2 c, and 2 d, page 87

Nicole

My family and I are looking forward to the future, actually. We're all upbeat about things. When I look at my kids, I see how much better off they are than I was at their age. By the time they get to be my age, they will have nailed down good jobs, they will have seen the world, they will have done all the things I wanted to do.

Martin

You watch the news today and it's all a bit of a downer, know what I mean? There's a degree of negativity that I never noticed in the past. By the end of this year we'll have had yet another election, but I don't see that making much of a difference. We just don't have politicians to give us the vision we're looking for.

Rose

I don't think anyone really believes that by year's end things will have gotten better. This time next year, employment won't have decreased, the environment won't have improved. Even now you look back, and all you see is a steady decline. It's depressing. I can't think of a time since I've been alive when things have gotten better, can you?

Edgar

Of course we have doubts about the future, but if you look at the past you see that bad times are always replaced by good. When I talk to my friends and neighbors—yes, they worry, they have their ups and downs, but basically they feel that things are on an upswing. That's the impression I get, anyway. Five years from now we'll all be better off; you just wait and see.

Tasks 3 a and 3 b, page 90

Male: Well, what do you think?

Female: Difficult. They're both very pleasant people—much better than the people we interviewed yesterday. And as project leaders they both have strengths.

M: And weaknesses.

F: Let's just take another look at what they had to say in the interview.

M: Well, Marty said he was looking for a new job because he wasn't named leader on the project he's currently working on, and he doesn't want to be on a team if he can't be a leader.

F: Angela isn't a team leader at the moment either.

M: But she said she doesn't mind being a team *member* sometimes. I also think that Angela's got enough motivation to finish a project without a lot of feedback, whereas Marty's boss said that he tends to drop the ball if he doesn't get constant praise.

F: On the other hand, Angela said that she would tend to do most of the work herself

if she thought that other people couldn't do it right.

M: While Marty has a good record of delegating tasks to other people.

F: Difficult, isn't it?

M: Mmm. One of the worries I have about Marty is his attitude. Technically, he's fine. I'm sure his project management skills are good, but I'm not sure that he'd be very good at accepting criticism. I think that his reaction would be one of anger—hostility even. Angela, on the other hand, would use criticism as a way of self-improvement.

F: I think you're right.

M: Another thing is their attitude toward people from different cultural backgrounds. That's an important consideration.

F: And they're both very strong in this area.

M: Yes, Angela's from an immigrant family herself, so she has first-hand experience of the challenges of settling in a new country.

F: And Marty's spent a great deal of his working life involved with immigrant communities.

M: So, who do we give it to?

F: Let's have a cup of coffee, and then I'll tell you who I think should get the job.

Unit 13 Time For a Change

Tasks 2 a, 2 b, and 2 c, page 95

Changes in my life? Well, I guess if I compare my life today with when I started working, there have been some pretty significant changes. In fact, things have changed so much over the years, it's difficult to know where to start. Let's see. When I started work, I used to ride a motorcycle. These days I drive to work in a car. I used to share a small apartment with three other guys, and we lived on macaroni and cheese! These days, I live in a decent house and eat in restaurants several nights a week. I remember the first vacation I took after I started work—I went surfing down the coast. Last year I went to a resort in Florida. I don't surf anymore, but I've just taken up golf. When I first started work, I had a girlfriend and married her the following year. Last year we got divorced. It was all very friendly, and we see each other quite often because of the kids.

Speaker 2: Changes? I guess the most important change in recent years would be Rick.

Questioner: Rick?

S: My boyfriend. We met, oh, about a year ago, I guess. I must say I wasn't very impressed with him when I first met him.

Q: You weren't.

S: No, I wasn't. We met at a mutual friend's party, and I thought he was loud and arrogant and opinionated. Well, he is, but he's also very intelligent and creative, so I guess that he has a right to be arrogant. Anyway, he thinks that I deserve him, because he asked me to marry him last week.

Q: Great! And what other important events have occurred in your life?

S: Other important events? Well, when I was fifteen I spent a year in Brazil.

Q: Brazil?

S: Yes, I went on a student exchange. It was fantastic, although I was terribly homesick.

Q: Where was that? Rio?

S: No. Recife. It's in the north—a fantastic place. And I guess looking back, going to school was significant. I went to a community college when I was eighteen, and had a pretty good time. Then getting this job last month was pretty significant to me. So, there you have it—work, relationships, education, and travel.

Q: And now you have the rest of your life to look forward to.

S: Uh, huh.

Task 1 a, page 97

Rick: What's up, Barbara?

Barbara: Oh, I don't know. I'm just in kind of a rut these days, I guess.

R: A rut?

B: Yeah. Same thing happens every day—there's nothing new going on.

R: That's too bad. Hey, there was something in yesterday's paper about how to get out of a rut. Let me find it for you.

B: You think it'll help me?

R: It might.

Task 4, page 98

Rick: Hi, Barbara!

Barbara: Oh, hi, Rick.

R: So, did that article help you any?

B: Rick, I really have to thank you for giving me that article to read. It really inspired me, and I decided that I was going to get out of my rut.

R: So what did you do?

B: Well, I'd always wanted to learn TypeRight. The word-processing program I've always used is EveryWord, and I thought this is my big opportunity to try something new.

R: And?

B: Well, I was supposed to have started next week in the Extension Program at Downtown Community College, but I waited too long to enroll, and when I finally called up the class was full.

R: Oh, no!

B: So I decided to take an art class instead—I've always wanted to learn watercolor painting.

R: Uh, huh.

B: Unfortunately, that didn't turn out too well

either—you wouldn't believe how expensive all the art supplies were—and they were *required* for class.

R: That's too bad.

B: Yeah. So, I decided, OK, I can always take up jogging. Unfortunately, I twisted my ankle the second time out. I thought the idea of playing tourist in my own town sounded like a great idea. I was supposed to have taken a walking tour last Saturday, but it rained all day.

R: You really have terrible luck.

B: You're not kidding. So, then I said, well, if I can't do anything for myself, I'll do something for others, and I volunteered to do library work at my sister's school, you know, working at the check-out desk. Trouble is, I'm supposed to have librarian training.

R: Even to do volunteer work?

B: Even to do volunteer work.

R: Well, I'm sorry things didn't work out.

B: Oh, I wouldn't say that.

R: You wouldn't?

B: No, all this running around has really gotten me out of my rut.

Unit 14 They're Only Words

Tasks 2 a and 2 b, page 102

Interviewer: I'm talking to linguistics professor Judith Baker about taboos. First of all, what does the word *taboo* actually mean?

Baker: Well, it comes from the South Sea Islands, where it means "holy" or "untouchable."

I: And taboos mainly exist in primitive societies, I guess.

B: Well, you might think that, but all societies have subjects they don't want to talk about, and there are taboos in sophisticated societies as well as primitive ones. Even in our super-sophisticated society it's believed that certain subjects are unlucky.

I: I see. And, ah, are there any subjects that are commonly avoided in different cultures?

B: Well, yes. There are differences, of course, but subjects such as the supernatural, sex, and death are considered taboo in many, many societies. Interestingly, animal names are also taboo in many different societies.

I: Animals?

B: Yes.

I: Could you give us some examples?

B: Sure. The Zuni Indians of New Mexico prohibit the use of the word for "frogs" during ceremonies. Here in the States I've heard people avoid using the word "bull" in polite speech, using "he cow" or "male beast" instead.

I: Really?

B: Yes. That was quite a few years ago now, but I did hear it. Other animal names that are taboo in various societies include wolves, weasels, rats, lice, and snakes. Further afield, there are even more extraordinary taboos. I came across a tribe of aborigines in Australia whose own names are taboo.

I: Their *own* names?

B: Yes. It's believed that if their name is even mentioned by another person something terrible will happen to them. So they have two names—a public name and a secret name.

I: Amazing. And how do we deal with taboos?

B: Well, the usual way is to find other words to replace the taboo ones. For example, in our society we have hundreds of ways of referring to death.

I: What, euphemisms like "passed away"?

B: Yes—"pass on," "go to rest." And some people use idioms like "kick the bucket" or "bite the dust."

Task 2 b, page 104

In our super-sophisticated society, it is believed that certain subjects are unlucky.

In many different societies, it is considered unlucky to mention animal names.

Among some Australian aboriginal tribes, it is believed that a person's name should never be used.

Among the Zuni Indians of New Mexico, it is prohibited to use the word for "frogs."

In parts of the United States, it is considered improper to use the word "bull."

Tasks 1 a and 1 b, page 105

Speaker: Hi, Charlie. Did you hear about the Wilson kid?

Charlie: I sure did. A four-month community service sentence and a three-thousand-dollar fine for spraying graffiti on the school wall. The judge said that he wanted to make an example of him. I think it's a disgrace.

S: So do I—defacing public property like that.

C: No, I mean it's a disgrace that he's being punished.

S: What?

C: I sympathize with the kid.

S: How can you say such a thing? He destroyed public property—the thing this country's built on. I believe that they should have put him away—a community service sentence is too soft. The kid's never been any good. I know him pretty well. He used to hang around with one of my kids till I put a stop to it.

C: Oh, come on. It isn't graffiti anyway; it's a very attractive wall mural. Let's face it, that old concrete wall was ugly before he painted it. When I'm waiting for my bus in the morning, I'd rather look at his painting than a dirty old wall.

S: Well, I disagree. I think it shows lack of respect for the values that have made this country great. Next thing he'll be spraying paint on cars. Besides, it's not even attractive—it's like some ugly piece of modern art.

C: And I bet you don't like modern art, right?

S: Right.

C: Well, I do, and I tell you, Dennis has got talent. And there are too few opportunities for artistic kids to find ways of expressing themselves these days. Doing murals is one way of letting them express themselves. It ought to be encouraged—in fact, they should be given paints for free and told to brighten the place up.

S: I'm afraid I just can't understand your attitude. As taxpayers, it's our money that's going to be used to clean up the mess. I, for one, am going to write a letter to the newspaper.

Unit 15 Review Unit

Task 3 a, page 110

Di: I guess I would have to say walking along the beach on a winter's day because of the peace and quiet and the smell of the salt and sea air.

Oh, it's a crazy one! I would really like to climb Mt. Everest—without oxygen. I saw a television program recently, and they did it from the bottom to the top of Mt. Everest without oxygen.

I think having a baby in my bathroom. I'd been to see the doctor two hours before and he said go away, the baby's not ready to be born yet, it'll come when it's ready. So I went home and all of a sudden it was ready, and I was in the bathroom having this baby all by myself.

Talking to some friends in a restaurant, and they left and I made some awful comment about their brat of a daughter, but I didn't realize the father had come back to get his jacket, which he'd left behind. She is a brat, but I wish he hadn't heard that.

The baby I had in the bathroom. Having him has changed my life. This really made me realize what's important.

Steve: Hmm. I guess lying on the floor after a hard day at the office, and listening to music on headphones. Mainly classical, but also blues and jazz.

I'd like to learn to paint. I collect modern art—nothing expensive or well-known, but nice to look at, you know. And I'd like to be able to do that myself.

Finishing a university degree, without a doubt. It took me years and years, but I did it in the end.

Let's see. I was in a bad car accident a few years ago and was almost killed. I broke my leg in five places and spent several weeks in the hospital. I'll never forget it.

A few years ago I went to the 30th anniversary concert for Bob Dylan in New York, and a friend of mine was involved in organizing the concert and I got invited to the party afterwards. It was fantastic—the concert and the party. I got to meet Dylan and all the other guitar heroes.

Unit 1 Celebrations

1B)

Example answers:
Sam: Hello, Melissa. This is Sam.
 I'm fine, thanks.
 Well, I got a letter from Kristin.
 She invited me to a Halloween party on Friday.
 Would you like to go with me?
 It doesn't start 'til nine.
 Do you think we have to dress up?
 I haven't decided yet.
 Could I collect you at 8:30?
 See you, Melissa, and thanks.

2.

movie/weird/porch/common/costumes/house-
holder/mean/yard/garbage/theory/practice/
parents.

3.

picture 1 = 3
        2 = 6
        3 = 1
        4 = 4
        5 = 2
        6 = 5

4A)

1. celebrate
2. commemorate
3. gift
4. ceremony
5. festival
6. elderly
7. invitation
8. tasteless
9. wedding
10. traditional

6.

1. Would you mind . . .
2. Can/Could/Would you be able to . . .
3. Would you mind . . .
4. Could/Can/Would you be able to . . .
5. Could/Can/Would you be able to . . .

Unit 2 Believe It or Not

1.

1. dramatic
2. explanation
3. recently
4. disbelief
5. believable
6. weirdest
7. coincidence
8. mysterious
9. superstitious
10. telepathic

2.

1. No, but I used to.
2. I'm sorry, I don't know how.
3. No, I didn't. Did you?
4. You're kidding.
5. No, never.

3.

1. when
2. where
3. where
4. why . . . where
5. how
6. why
7. how
8. when

4A)

Example notes:
   Because he heard a loud noise and wanted to investigate.
   Bright lights and a space craft above the house.
   He felt he had to.

They had large heads and thin arms and legs. They were short with large eyes.

Spacious and comfortable, all white, and the floors and walls were soft.

He took a taxi.

Excited, not frightened.

Through telepathy.

Disbelief.

5.

4, 3, 1, 2, 7, 11, 5, 6, 10, 9, 8

Unit 3 Origins

1. Example notes:

Sudden job offer teaching in Mexico. Had written applying for job in the summer, but didn't even get a reply. One of the institute teachers broke his contract, so I was offered the job. Had to leave in a hurry.

First apartment no good. He wanted a Mexican landlady, not a Dane. Also no good because he's allergic to cats. Has now found great apartment downtown—Mexican colonial style. Right size, right price.

All Mexican students—same language problems. Easier then teaching multi-national classes.

Mexican food—delicious.

2A)

1. Malcom Stephenson.
2. She thinks it's cool.
3. Brighton/a town near London.
4. A year ago.
5. No.
6. A castle.
7. Four days ago.
8. Julia.
9. No.
10. It's very cosmopolitan.

3.

```
T                       I
O                       D
L                       E
E                       N         O
R                       T         R
A   N A T I O N A L I T I E S
N           P         T         G
C           P         Y         I
E           U             I
        C U L T U R E     N
            A         M   S E T T L E M E N T S
            T             I M M I G R A T I O N
            I         G
            O         R
            N         A
                      T
                  D E V E L O P M E N T
                      D
```

1. tolerance
2. nationalities
3. population
4. identity
5. origins
6. culture
7. settlements
8. emigrated
9. immigration
10. development

4.

1. have never lived
2. liked
3. has read
4. have never heard
5. went . . . read
6. have known . . . was
7. have settled
8. stopped . . . didn't wake
9. moved . . . have never regretted
10. have been

Unit 4 Good Advice

1.

  1. workaholic
  2. physician
  3. quit
  4. deep
  5. busy
  6. nap
  7. exercise
  8. ritual
  9. regular
10. turkey
11. mattress

  1. down = acupuncture

2.

  1. who
  2. whose
  3. who
  4. whose
  5. who's
  6. who
  7. who's
  8. whose

5. For example:
You should teach your family to get their own breakfast.
If things get stressful at work, you should take a short break.
If your boss asks you to take work home, you should tell her that you can't work weekends.
Whenever possible, you should have a sit-down lunch.
When your husband is home, you should get him to help you.

6.
He mentions 1, 5, 6.
Lori says he should take something of theirs when next they borrow something of his, or he should keep his closets locked.

Unit 5 Review

2.
whose, What, in, at, who, to, for, during, where, After, should.

3.
  1. . . . that makes this ice cream so good.
  2. . . . if I brought Sergio to the party?
  3. . . . get a taxi if you miss the bus.
  4. . . . to share a house with someone who smokes.
  5. . . . eaten since 10 A.M. yesterday.

5.
  1. Have . . . seen
  2. read
  3. Did . . . go
  4. have lived
  5. haven't heard
  6. predicted

7.
  1. cure
  2. drown
  3. spooky
  4. refugee
  5. festival
  6. disbelief
  7. caffeine
  8. tossing
  9. origin
10. sense
11. neat

Unit 6 That's a Smart Idea

1A) For example:

This person is having trouble with her youngest son, who is 17. He doesn't study, and he spends hours on the phone. He gets angry when asked to hang up.

Her husband, who's a doctor, needs the phone line to be free because his patients call him. Her eldest son, who's a journalist, also needs to use the phone. They can't afford to pay the telephone bill.

3.
1. . . . was written in her favorite purple ink.
2. . . . were written by a little known British writer in the nineteenth century.
3. . . . has been composed about one man's search for world peace.
4. . . . last movie was admired by the critics.
5. . . . have been offered a job as a newscaster for a major TV network.

4A) For example:

She said she had a bad cough. She said her throat was sore and her cough was so bad that she couldn't sleep at night. She told the doctor that she hated it when she didn't sleep well, because she had to get up early in the morning. She said she had to make breakfast for her children and take them to school. She told him that was why she had decided to come and see him.

4B)

Teacher: Your essay's quite interesting. You've obviously done a lot of reading about the subject, but you've made a lot of careless mistakes in spelling and punctuation.

5A)

29/*Girl with Hairbrush*/1993/Gershwode

5B)
1. He wanted to show youth and maturity.
2. He said he didn't like it, and he thought it was unsuccessful. It made him think he was in the middle of a green salad.
3. She liked it. She said it made her feel calm and relaxed.

6.
1. writer
2. musician
3. dentist
4. songwriter
5. architect

7.
1. Scrub
2. warn
3. Sprinkle
4. pour
5. store

Unit 7 Creatures Great and Small

1.

reptiles/dinosaurs/species/endangered/magical/spring/lay/hole/crabs/habitat/extinct

2.
1. Penguins are birds that can't fly.
2. Turtles are reptiles whose shells are hard.
3. Reptiles are animals whose blood is cold.
4. Elephants are animals that live in groups.
5. Whales are mammals whose young are born in the water.
6. The Atticus Atlas is a butterfly that measures 9¾ inches across the wings.
7. Chimpanzees are animals whose offspring remain dependent for four or five years.
8. Bears are mammals that hibernate in the winter.

3. For example:

It is the most delicious ice cream I have ever tasted.

It's the worst joke I've ever heard.

She's the most unusual person I've ever met.

It's the biggest dog I've ever seen.

It's the most dramatic photo he's ever taken.

4.

1. About $10 billion a year.
2. private collectors, pet shops, zoos, circuses, and for medical research
3. apes/sea turtles/giant pandas/cheetahs/Asian elephants/leopards
4. For example: For every animal on sale, hundreds die.
   The cruelty involved in trapping and transporting the animals.
5. For example: Birds are force-fed before being transported.
   Birds are packed tight into spare tires or boxes with no room to move.
6. Control the consumers.

5A)

1. . . . his wife wanted a dog.
2. 10
3. . . . worried about . . .
4. . . . doesn't have . . .

5B)

1. . . . a local pet store.
2. . . . he loved her.
3. . . . means "illusion" in Hindi.
4. . . . he kept the dog.
5. . . . she seemed to be in pain when she walked.
6. . . . he dedicated all his time to her.
7. . . . to put her to sleep and get on with his life.
8. . . . his behavior.

Unit 8 Communications

1A)

1. confirmed
2. postpone
3. comparing
4. recommend
5. valuable
6. incompetent
7. difficult
8. convince
9. fax
10. quality
11. intentions
12. solution
13. plan
14. distinctive
15. down = communications

3A)

RELATIONSHIP NOW

his hair, his clothes, his earring, his friends, the places he goes, how he spends his time, the music he listens to.

RELATIONSHIP IN THE PAST

used to have a great time together, were always together, went shopping together, ate together, enjoyed same TV programs, talked all the time.

4.

1. give up
2. put up with
3. putting . . . off
4. cut down
5. planning on
6. take up
7. looks forward to
8. keep on

5A)

Greg White

Tanya King

A three-bedroom house

In Lake View

Almost new, recently painted

$175,000

Tomorrow morning

5B) For example:

Caller: I wonder if you could put me through to extension 415.

Secretary: I'm afraid that line is busy at the moment.

Caller: Could you tell me when I could speak to Mr. Bridge?

Secretary: It won't be possible this morning.

Caller: Do you think you could ask him if he's free this afternoon?

Secretary: Yes . . . he will be free this afternoon.

Caller: I wonder if you would tell him that Karen Lindt will be coming to speak to him about the Civic Center project?

Secretary: Yes, of course.

Unit 9 Helping Hands

1.

1. sign
2. award
3. causes
4. sponsor
5. attorney
6. highlight
7. donation
8. charity
9. Famine
10. raise
11. cash

2.

1. It gives mobility to paralyzed people.
2. He was going to play football professionally.
3. To regain his independence.
4. He wanted to share his feeling of liberation with others.

2A)

1. discouraging, causing a loss of hope and confidence.
2. unable to move.
3. turns around quickly.
4. not easy to notice.
5. without feeling.
6. makes the car go in a particular direction.
7. skillfully.
8. hold.

2B) For example:

He wouldn't have started "Get Mobile" if he hadn't lost the use of his arms and legs.

He wouldn't have got on with his life if his family hadn't supported him.

If he had broken his neck higher up, he wouldn't have been able to drive again.

If he had felt sorry for himself, he wouldn't have become independent again.

3A)

CRISTINA LOPEZ:

Left paralyzed after an accident. Unable to leave her house.

Uses van once a week. Got her freedom back.

MABEL GRANT:

Her husband is brain damaged, paralyzed, and in a hospital. She wants to take him out sometimes.

Can take him once a week to a park, the beach, or the mall.

THE PIKE FAMILY:

Son is a quadriplegic. Couldn't go on a family holiday.

With "Get Mobile" van, could go camping in mountains for two weeks.

How you can help: By sending a donation.

What money will be spent on: Adapting new van.

Where to send money: P.O. Box 507, Westport (or call 866-3490).

4.
1. . . . had got up on time, I wouldn't have missed the bus.
2. . . . to help us to help them.
3. . . . to give generously.
4. . . . have burned down if I hadn't extinguished the fire.
5. . . . to talk to their friends about the Aid Appeal.
6. . . . have donated something if she hadn't been rude.
7. . . . to work together.
8. . . . have caught a cold if he hadn't gone out in the rain.

Unit 10 Review

2.
1. . . . has . . . had?
2. . . . was designed . . .
3. . . . would have donated . . .
4. . . . was cancelled . . .
5. . . . have . . . seen.
6. . . . were taken . . .
7. . . . had been . . .
8. . . . was killed . . .

3. 1. . . . I was planning for the following weekend.

2. . . . that have cold blood/whose blood is cold.
3. . . . up with your lateness anymore.
4. . . . Jane had told him about it the day before.
5. . . . forward to going to the film festival.
6. . . . if I wanted those books.
7. . . . off going to the dentist.
8. . . . if you could lend me your mobile phone?
9. . . . his brother ran a small direct-mail business from home.
10. . . . you to take a few minutes to read this.

4. For example:
I would have turned the gas off before leaving the kitchen.

I wouldn't have left the ice cream in the shopping bag.

I would have remembered to put water in the vase.

I wouldn't have left the steaks where the dog could get them.

I would have invited my friends out to a restaurant.

5.
1. precious
2. homeless
3. voicemail
4. mammals
5. sprinkled
6. shattered
7. plan
8. buzzer
9. keep
10. petition

1. down = chimpanzee

Unit 11 Speaking Personally

1A)
1. Seeing her book published.
2. Listening to her grandmother read her stories.
3. To write a movie script.
4. Traveling.
5. Moving to her new house on the beach.

2.

ACROSS	DOWN
1. impatient	1. influential
2. do	2. easygoing
3. deny	3. résumé
4. intense	4. avoid
5. ambition	5. doing
6. intend	

3A)

POSITIVE

clever, obedient, reliable, sincere, responsible, neat, fair, capable, confident, mature, happy

NEGATIVE

clumsy, arrogant, cold, nervous, mean, indecisive, stupid, cruel

3B)

-ty:
reliability, sincerity, responsibility, maturity, capability
-nce:
obedience, confidence, arrogance
-ness:
cleverness, neatness, fairness, clumsiness, coldness, nervousness, meanness, indecisiveness

4A)

His father was head ranger of a reserve in Kenya. Animals always part of his life.

Made a film about lions. Sequence with birth of lion cubs. Won an award.

Film about mountain gorillas. Took two years. Most exciting experience.

A film about koala bears in Australia.

4B)
1. . . . was almost more important to me than being with people.
2. . . . took longer than all the rest of the film.
3. . . . is the easiest part of the job.
4. . . . we would have lost the film and probably our lives.
5. . . . was the most exciting experience of my career.

5.
1. How did you avoid laughing at the joke?
2. When do you expect to graduate?
3. Why did you suggest going to the doctor?
4. How could you deny crashing the car?
5. I enjoy playing tennis on Sundays.
6. What do you want to do this afternoon?
7. What types of activities do you dislike doing most?
8. When do you hope to arrive?

Unit 12 Attitudes

1. optimist, turn, upbeat, by, prediction, off, next, opportunities, standard, have, attitude, potential

2. By the end of the month she will have hired the chef. . . .

. . . she will have interviewed and hired the waiters.

. . . she will have gotten the permit from the fire department.

. . . she will have bought the furniture.

. . . she will have paid the decorator.

. . . she will have checked the kitchen equipment.

. . . she will have sent invitations for the grand opening.

3A)
1. . . . shouldn't I?
2. . . . has she?
3. . . . did you?
4. . . . didn't she?
5. . . . won't you?

4A)
1. 92 days.
2. To save a two-hundred-year-old tree.
3. By pretending to be reporters and requesting an interview.
4. He thinks we must act. We must take responsibility and fight for what we believe in.
5. About the police impersonating journalists.
6. He was unconcerned, because it was legal.
7. Because the tree will have been cut down by the time he is released.

5.
3, 5, 1, 4, 2, 9, 6, 7, 10, 8 (Nelson Mandela)

Unit 13 Time For a Change

1A)
1. dependent 2. significant 3. rut
4. experience 5. expectations 6. leisure
7. predictable 8. sample
9. vary 10. help

1B)
1. rut 2 dependent 3. help 4. leisure
5. significant 6. sample 7. expectations
8. predictable 9. vary 10. experience

2.
1. She couldn't decide what to do with her life, and she floated into it.
2. She didn't feel any real vocation for it.
3. She washed her clothes and bought food for the week. She ironed, and she chose a video to watch on Sunday evening.
4. Because the school principal asked her to. She thought it was a specialized job.
5. Nothing in the class was predictable. She had to work hard and be imaginative. It made her feel she had a talent for teaching. It was a change.

4.
has been seeing/are going/have . . . joined/have been visiting/read/had . . . heard/told/protecting/had . . . attended/has been spending

5.
1. When she was about 12.
2. Read books and listen to the radio.
3. Three or four hours every night.
4. 21.
5. He's traveled on planes many times.
6. Man's first walk on the moon.
7. Read a book about it.
8. Because times have changed since his grandmother was young.

Unit 14 They're Only Words

1.
1. credibility
2. popularity
3. prohibit
4. check
5. indecisive
6. humorous
7. graffiti

8. sarcastic
9. demand
10. down = graffiti

2.
1. It was his birthday.
2. It was his favorite breakfast.
3. A hat. She thought it was time he started to wear one.
4. A baseball cap. They thought it would keep the sun off his head.
5. A ski cap. She said it was to keep his head warm.
6. "You're getting a bit thin on top."
7. You're going bald.

4A)
1. . . . believed that black cats are unlucky.
2. . . . said that many popular festivals have religious origins.
3. . . . is maintained that children shouldn't express their own opinions in front of adults.
4. . . . is believed that hearing certain music can cure sickness.
5. . . . sometimes assumed that changing your lifestyle will change your luck.

4B) a. . . . having second thoughts . . .
     b. . . . throwing her weight around . . .
     c. . . . bite my tongue . . .
     d. . . . hit it off . . .
     e. . . . snap out of it . . .

5.
1. Because Eric told Zac he could go to a party.
2. Zac has an exam.
3. He'll be too tired to study.
4. Nearly 18.
5. You can't always keep him tied to your apron strings.

6. She says he'll destroy his credibility as a role model.

Unit 15 Review

1. For example:
1. Adam went to the mailbox to check his mail, didn't he?
2. He didn't get to class on time, did he?
3. He's an economics student, isn't he?
4. His parents had given him a car, hadn't they?
5. You don't need lots of money to be happy, do you?
6. Adam was dreaming, wasn't he?
7. He could re-enroll in college later, couldn't he?
8. Adam has a positive attitude, doesn't he?

2.
1. rut
2. workout
3. talented
4. competitive
5. euphemism
6. uphold
7. credibility
8. achievement
9. delegate

3.
. . . don't you?
. . . wasn't he?
. . . didn't he?
. . . has lost . . .
. . . began . . .
. . . was walking . . .
. . . came . . .
. . . had never seen . . .
. . . unfolded . . .
. . . had gone . . .

...had lost...
...had been looking...
...had dreamed...
...decided...
...was offered...
...has been working...
...has lived...
...hasn't smoked...
...has gotten...
...has eaten...
...married...
...isn't it?
...won't you?

4.
1. bite her tongue
2. give them a piece of my mind
3. hit it off
4. snap out of it
5. have second thoughts
6. bend over backwards

5.
1. ...thought rude to interrupt.
2. ...to help us.
3. ...have been married for 20 years.
4. ...going to the beach.
5. ...is thought perfectly normal for men to wear earrings.
6. ...to have called Julie.
7. ...to buy flowers.
8. ...will have lost my job.
9. ...been working with Wiley and Hogan for four years.

Unit 1 Celebrations

Task 3, page 3

You will need a large pumpkin. Cut off the top and hollow out the flesh with a sharp knife. Be careful not to cut yourself. Pumpkins are very hard on the outside, and the knife could easily slip. Now it's time to shape the eyes. It's easiest if you cut out triangles where the eyes should be. When you've finished the eyes, cut out a line of triangles for the teeth. Stand a candle inside the pumpkin. A short, broad candle is best because it won't fall over easily. Now your jack-o'-lantern is ready. Put it on your porch, and don't forget—light the candle as soon as it gets dark.

Unit 2 Believe It or Not

Task 4 a, page 7

Wife: Where on earth have you been? I've been worried sick.

Husband: You're not going to believe me.

Wife: Try me. What happened?

Husband: Well, soon after you left I heard a loud noise, like a helicopter trying to land. I went out of the house to see what it was. There were lots of bright lights—and I could see a large object directly above the house. It was some sort of space craft.

Wife: You're kidding.

Husband: I knew you wouldn't believe me. Well, then the object moved off north, and I just had this compulsion to follow it. I got into the car and drove, keeping it in sight all the time. It kept ahead of me, pretty high up in the sky, and then all of a sudden it came down by the side of the car. A door opened, and framed in the doorway I could see this alien figure . . .

Wife: Give me a break!

Husband: *(ignoring her)* It motioned me to come, and I got out of the car and before I knew it, I was inside the craft.

Wife: I suppose you went traveling around the universe, and I suppose the aliens had large heads and antennae.

Husband: They had large heads and thin arms and legs. They were pretty small—about half of my height, and they had large eyes. No antennae, though. There were six of them. We communicated through telepathy.

Wife: *(slightly hostile)* Oh, really. I find that hard to believe.

Husband: I didn't feel at all frightened. In fact, it was very exciting and the craft was spacious and comfortable, all white. No furniture, but the walls and floor were soft. I don't know where we traveled—there were no windows and there was no sensation of movement.

Wife: *(in disbelief)* You're really serious, aren't you? You really think this happened?

Husband: Yes, it really happened. It seemed like a very short time and I suddenly found myself back where I left the car. Only the car wasn't there, so I took a taxi home, and here I am!

Wife: I just can't believe it, Tom. Now tell me what really happened . . .

Unit 3 Origins

Task 2 a, page 11

Julia: Hi.

Malcolm: Hello.

Julia: I'm Julia.

Malcolm: Nice to meet you, Julia. I'm Malcolm—Malcolm Stephenson.

Julia: Isn't this a great party, Malcolm? I think this music's really cool!

Malcolm: Yes, it is a good party.

Julia: Hey! You're British, aren't you?

Malcolm: Well, yes I am, actually.

Julia: I was in London last year. Do you come from London?

Malcolm: No. I come from a town called Brighton—it's quite near London.

Julia: Oh, yeah? I've been there. I went there on the same trip. We visited some sort of castle on the coast, I think. Would that be right?

Malcolm: Yes! Brighton Pavilion.

Julia: How are you enjoying New York?

Malcolm: Hard to say, I've only been here for four days. I arrived on Wednesday. Anyway, I'm enjoying it so far. And there's so much to see, isn't there? So much going on . . .

Julia: I've always been fascinated by British culture. I've read lots of books about life in Britain. That's why I went. I wanted to see it for myself.

Malcolm: And what did you think of the British?

Julia: I hardly ever saw any. I met many more Indians, Pakistanis, Spaniards, West Indians, and Arabs than British people while I was in London. And that goes for most of the other places I visited in Britain, too!

Malcolm: Yes. It's very cosmopolitan. That's what I like about it. It's just like New York in that respect.

Unit 4 Good Advice

Task 6, page 18

Lori: Jeff, it's freezing out here. For goodness sake, put a sweater on.

Jeff: I can't. I don't have one.

Lori: What on earth do you mean? You must have a sweater!

Jeff: Well, not one that's available at the moment. It's the kids, you see. Danny borrowed the thick green one, Peter has my short red one—the one you gave me for my birthday—and Susan was wearing the gray one when I saw her leave the house this morning. The brown one with the black buttons—that disappeared from my closet last week, and nobody seems to know where it is.

Lori: Good heavens! Don't they have their own sweaters?

Jeff: Yes, of course they do, but . . . although they are smart kids with good grades at school, they don't seem to grasp the concept of personal property. I keep telling them, "This belongs to me. Please don't move it or touch it without my permission," but I might as well be talking to the wall. Nothing of mine is safe. My razor, my cologne, my clothes, my pens, my CDs. Their rule seems to be "Use it, destroy it, but never put it back where you found it." This morning it was my silk shirt. "OK, who borrowed it?" I said. "Not me," they all answered. They all had such a look of innocence and surprise!

Lori: Jeff, drastic action is what is called for. You have spoiled your children shamelessly. You shouldn't allow it! When they borrow something of yours next time you should . . . you should . . . er . . . go to their rooms and take something of theirs! If they don't learn to respect your things, you should get a key to your closets and keep them locked . . . you should . . .

Jeff: Ah, there goes Susan with my gray sweater. I must say she looks good in it. Susan! . . . Susan . . .

Unit 6 That's a Smart Idea

Task 5, page 28

Man: What's the title of that painting?

Woman: Let me see. Number twenty-nine . . . *Girl with Hairbrush*.

Man: What? I can't see a hairbrush.

Woman: And I can't see a girl.

Man: When was it painted?

Woman: Er . . . 1993.

Man: Who was it painted by?

Woman: A man called Gershwode. G-E-R-S-H-W-O-D-E. It says he wanted to show youth and maturity.

Man: Well, he failed. All I can see is a lot of green paint.

Woman: In the catalog it says Gershwode's use of green paint symbolizes youth.

Man: Well, I can't see it, and I don't like the painting at all. It makes me think that I'm in the middle of a green salad. What do you think?

Woman: I think you're very intolerant. Yes, I think I do like it. It certainly doesn't make me think of a green salad. I think it makes me feel sort of calm and relaxed.

Unit 7 Creatures Great and Small

Task 4, page 31

Radio Host: Today on the program we are going to talk about the illegal trade in live wild animals, and to tell us more about it is Janet Jones, who is an animal activist and author of a book on the subject, *Cruel Passage*, published just last week. Janet, what can you tell us about this illegal trade?

Janet: This is a shameful and scandalous trade. Nobody can know for sure, but experts calculate that it is worth $10 billion a year. Birds, mammals, reptiles, and fish are taken from their natural habitat and sold to private collectors, pet shops, zoos, circuses, and also for medical research. There is a great demand for exotic animals, many of them endangered—apes, sea turtles, giant pandas, cheetahs, and Asian elephants, to name only a few. People will pay enormous sums for them. A baby leopard, for example, brings $4,600. And the most terrible thing is that we are killing the masterpieces of life on the planet, all because of our greed and ignorance.

Host: In your book you talk of environmental devastation and the enormous cruelty of the trade. Can you give us some examples of this?

Janet: Yes. For every animal on sale, hundreds die. Part of the problem is the primitive methods of trapping. Poachers kill mother apes to get their young. Tropical bird trappers use hidden nets and snares so flocks of birds fly into them. The unwanted or injured birds are left to die. To capture tropical fish, poachers spray poison into coral waters. The poison stuns but does not kill the fish, and then it is easy to collect the creatures, but the poison remains, killing the fragile coral reefs. Trappers cut down trees to get baby birds in their high nests—the loss of habitat is devastating. And the cruelty is incredible. Birds, which make up the largest portion of the contraband, are often force-fed before shipment. Then, with their wings clipped and their beaks forced shut, they are packed tight into spare tires, handbags, or boxes, with no room to move. The majority of birds die before they reach their destination. One of the most pathetic sights I have ever seen was a box of 200 birds, all of them dead. Every one of them had died on the journey.

Host: What, if anything, can be done?

Janet: The best thing is to control the consumers—the buyers, not the sellers. Nobody needs a pet tiger. Nobody needs a pet monkey. Exotic animals are wonderfully inspiring, but it's best to see them in nature, not in zoos.

Unit 8 Communications

Task 5 a, page 38

Mrs. King: Hello.

Man: Good morning. I believe you're selling a three-bedroom house.

Mrs. King: That's correct.

Man: Could you tell me where the house is?

Mrs. King: Sure. It's in Lake View.

Man: Lake View. That sounds nice. How far from the lake is it?

Mrs. King: Oh, it overlooks the lake. It has the most wonderful view.

Man: Really? That sounds great. I wonder if you could tell me what condition the house is in?

Mrs. King: It's practically new. We only built it two years ago. But I just got a new job, and we have to move away from the area. And we had the house completely repainted before putting it onto the market.

Man: Would you tell me how much you're asking for the house?

Mrs. King: We had the house valued at $175,000, so that's what we're hoping to get.

Man: Do you think I could come and see the house this afternoon?

Mrs. King: This afternoon's a bit difficult.

Man: How about tomorrow?

Mrs. King: What time do you think you could come?

Man: At about eleven o'clock in the morning.

Mrs. King: Yes. I think that would be fine.

Man: OK. Until eleven o'clock tomorrow then. And thank you very much.

Mrs. King: Oh, what's your name?

Man: Greg . . . Greg White. And yours?

Mrs. King: Tanya King.

Man: See you tomorrow, Mrs. King.

Unit 9 Helping Hands

Task 3 a, page 42

Announcer's Voice: And now a local radio appeal on behalf of "Get Mobile." Cristina

Lopez was a nurse at Bridgetown Hospital in 1988. While on the night shift, she slipped on a wet floor in the hospital and broke her neck. She was left paralyzed, and for two years she was unable to leave her house, except when she went to doctor's appointments in a transport van.

Cristina: My life was changed when I saw an ad for "Get Mobile." I was confined to a wheelchair and had been unable to get out and about for two years. But through "Get Mobile" I now have access to a van once a week. The people at "Get Mobile" taught me how to drive it. It's wonderful. It's like getting your freedom back. I am able to go shopping again, visit friends, go out to dinner. It's the most wonderful feeling of liberation.

Announcer: Mabel Grant's husband was left brain damaged and paralyzed after a series of operations. He is now being cared for in a hospital. Mabel wanted to be able to take him out occasionally, but until recently this was impossible.

Mabel: Now I collect a "Get Mobile" van once a week. I am so grateful to be able to take my husband out in his wheelchair on weekends. We go for the day to a park, or to the beach, and sometimes to the mall. It's the time of the week we both look forward to.

Announcer: The Pike family's dream was to go on a camping trip together. A simple enough dream, but for the Pike family it was difficult to fulfill, because their son is a quadriplegic.

Mr. Pike: Luke, our youngest son, is disabled and confined to a wheelchair, so getting away on a family vacation is a real problem. Through "Get Mobile" we were able to have a van for two weeks last summer and go up into the mountains with our tent. This was a special time for all of us, one we will always treasure, and we could never have done it without "Get Mobile."

Announcer: For five years now, "Get Mobile," a nonprofit organization, has been dedicated to giving back mobility to the physically disabled in the Westport area. We need your help. Your donation would go toward making the necessary adaptations to the new van we have just bought. Please send your check to P.O. Box 507, Westport, or call 866-3490 for more information. Thank you.

Unit 11 Speaking Personally

Tasks 4 a and 4 b, pages 52 and 53

Interviewer: Pete, you've been making documentaries about wild animals for the last twenty years. What led you to this career, or did you fall into it by accident?

Pete: It was certainly no accident. I grew up surrounded by wild animals, and they've always fascinated me. My father was the head ranger of a reserve in Kenya, so wild animals were always part of my life. In fact, being with animals was almost more important to me than being with people.

Interviewer: I believe you won an award for the first documentary you ever made.

Pete: Yes, it was about lions. We filmed the birth of some lion cubs. Getting that sequence took longer than all the rest of the film. We had to build a special shelter where we could film from, but where the lions couldn't see or smell us. We spent days inside. It was very uncomfortable. But often filming the animals is the easiest part of the job. On that occasion, after we had finished filming and were heading back to civilization, we ran into some poachers. It was a nasty situation, and I'm sure they were planning to kill us and take our equipment. But we were lucky. Some rangers arrived just in time. If they hadn't turned up, we would have lost the film and probably our lives.

Interviewer: Tell me about your most recent film.

Pete: It's about mountain gorillas. It took me two years to make, and I think it's my greatest achievement so far. Living with those noble creatures was the most exciting experience of my career.

Interviewer: What are the qualities that make a good wildlife photographer?

Pete: Well, you certainly need to be patient. It could take days to get any footage that is worthwhile. You need to be persistent and dedicated. Living for months in uncomfortable places, with only one or two other people for company, is not everyone's idea of fun.

Interviewer: And for your next project?

Pete: Well, I intend to make a film about koala bears. In fact, I'm leaving for Australia next week.

Unit 12 Attitudes

Task 4 a, page 56

Julius Grant, arrested this morning by police posing as journalists, talked of his three-month protest to save a tree believed to be two hundred years old. The protester, looking tired but vowing to continue the fight, explained that he had spent 92 days in the branches of the tree in order to prevent it from being chopped down to make way for the construction of a shopping mall. Police said Tuesday that they had used "a bit of cunning" to make the arrest. Police Officer Baines explained that he and another officer, pretending they were reporters, had requested an interview. The activist, deceived by the false identification badges, pulled them up into the tree, where the officers grabbed him around the throat, handcuffed him, and then lowered him to the ground.

Julius Grant later told reporters that it was a disgrace that the authorities were allowing the destruction of the two-hundred-year-old oak: "We are destroying our environment in the name of progress. I believe it is the responsibility of each of us to fight for what we believe in. Words are not enough. We must act." Asked what he thought he had achieved by the protest, Grant said, "I'm optimistic that my actions will encourage others to fight for a better future, to save our planet from the short-sighted actions of fools."

Meanwhile, local journalists lodged a complaint to the police about the impersonation, but Officer Baines was unconcerned. He said that it was legal for police to impersonate journalists, but not for journalists to impersonate police.

A spokesperson for the construction company building the shopping mall said the tree will have been cut down by the time Grant is released from custody Sunday.

Unit 13 Time For a Change

Task 5, page 63

Tommy: Have things changed a lot since you were young, Grandma?

Grandmother: Oh, they certainly have, Tommy. You would be surprised.

Tommy: How?

Grandmother: Well, for one thing, not everybody had a television when I was young. We didn't have one in our house until I was roundabout twelve.

Tommy: What did you do?

Grandmother: We listened to the radio and read books, of course.

Tommy: I read books.

Grandmother: Yes, but you don't read books like I read books. I was expected to read three or four hours every night.

Tommy: And did you?

Grandmother: Usually . . . not always.

Tommy: What else was different?

Grandmother: Well, there were planes, but not everybody traveled on them, like they do today. I was twenty-one before I had ever been on an airplane, as a matter of fact.

Tommy: I've traveled on planes millions of times.

Grandmother: Well, that's a bit of an exaggeration, but anyway things are very different now.

Tommy: What was the most exciting thing that ever happened when you were young?

Grandmother: Let me see . . . Oh, yes. The most exciting thing must have been when man first walked on the moon. We all watched it on television.

Tommy: Tell me about it.

Grandmother: I'll do better than that. I'll lend you a book about it. You can read it before you go to bed.

Tommy: Oh, Grandma.

Grandmother: Remember, when I was young I was supposed to read three or four hours before I went to sleep.

Tommy: Yes. Well, times have changed now!

Unit 14 They're Only Words

Task 5, page 68

Rosemary: Eric, is that you?

Eric: Yes. Hello, Rosemary.

Rosemary: Why did you tell Zac he could go out late to a party tonight? You know he's got an exam on Monday.

Eric: Rosemary, it's only a party. He can study tomorrow.

Rosemary: You know perfectly well that if he goes to a party tonight, he won't come home until two or three in the morning. He'll be much too tired to study tomorrow.

Eric: He promised me he would be home by one o'clock!

Rosemary: Oh, really, Eric. I just can't understand your attitude. Zac never comes home early on Friday nights. He'll forget his promise to you before he's even reached the end of the road.

Eric: Oh, come on, Rosemary. Zac isn't like that. He's a very responsible person.

Rosemary: No, he isn't. He's no more responsible than any other person his age.

Eric: Well, I disagree with you. And Zac's nearly eighteen now. You've got to let go of him a bit. You can't always keep him tied

to your apron strings. He's far too dependent on you as it is.

Rosemary: How can you say such a thing? Zac
pays no attention to me at all. And he's
always going to parties—you know he is.

Eric: Listen, Rosemary, I have to get back to
work. We'll talk about this when I get
home tonight.

Rosemary: OK. But you have to be firm with
Zac, or else you'll destroy your credibility
as a role model.

Eric: All right . . . all right. We'll talk about it
tonight. Good-bye!